25 WAYS TO CURE THE HICCUPS:

UNCOVERING THE TRUTH BEHIND

101 COMMON MYTHS AND MISCONCEPTIONS

BRIAN UDERMANN, Ph. D.

D1042940

TEST YOUR KNOWLEDGE

BEFORE YOU BEGIN reading this book I would like to encourage you to test your knowledge on the myths that are included in the following pages. Read through the table of contents starting on the next page and indicate whether you think each myth is true or false by checking the appropriate box. For an added twist, sit down with your spouse, a parent, sibling, or a friend and go through them together. After reading the book, go through and count how many you got right. Look for your score below to see where your knowledge level is in regard to common myths and misconceptions.

SCORE	KNOWLEDGE
90 or above	Excellent
80 to 89	Very Good
70 to 79	Good
60 to 69	Fair
59 or below	Consider reading the book twice

TABLE OF CONTENTS

Section Three: General Health 93   T or F?

ACKNOWLEDGEMENTS

I WOULD LIKE to start by thanking my wife and three children. I have been blessed with a truly wonderful family, and spending time with them constantly reminds me of what is really important in life. I love to speak on the topic of myths and misconceptions, and many of the stories I tell are from our family adventures.

I'd also like to thank Jen Holman, a librarian at the University of Wisconsin-La Crosse. Jen helped find research studies for some of the myths and was often able to locate articles when I wasn't able to.

Finally, I'd like to thank my parents. Even though my mother and father didn't go to school after the 8th grade, they instilled in me a thirst for knowledge and learning that is still active and alive today. They both taught me the importance of having a strong work ethic and that you should always treat people with respect.

INTRODUCTION

A QUICK INTERNET search will reveal hundreds, maybe even thousands, of ways people attempt to "cure" their hiccups. Here are twenty-five strategies that I have heard people say work:

Burp • Laugh • Cough • Gargle • Chew gum • Eat mustard • Eat chocolate • Drink vinegar • Suck on a lemon • Hold your breath • Drink pickle juice • Take a hot shower • Rub your ear lobe • Hang upside down • Stand on your head • Drink Tabasco sauce • Blow on your thumb • Drink a glass of water • Eat a spoonful of sugar • Have someone scare you • Immerse your face in ice water • Ask someone to tickle you • Eat a tablespoon of peanut butter • Pull on your tongue with your thumb and index finger

My personal favorite is a combination of two of the above: Stand on your head while drinking a glass of water. If you can do that, you are truly talented!

Extensive research in my house involving three children, a teaspoon, and a bowl of sugar has shown the spoonful of sugar remedy is a sure-fire cure, most of the time anyway. As silly as some of these remedies sound, it's likely that we've all tried some of them and swear by at least one.

I first started getting interested in myths and misconceptions when I was teaching a health and wellness course to university students. As I was covering topics like cardiovascular health, muscular fitness, flexibility, behavior change, aerobic exercise, and body fat, I started including two or three myths on those topics in each lecture. I could tell right away that the students really enjoyed hearing and learning about the myths, probably because many of the things their parents or other people had told them were not true. I then decided to create a standalone lecture on myths and misconceptions. It was pretty remarkable how much students enjoyed learning about the various myths I was covering. In fact, one semester I surveyed my students and asked them which lecture from the entire course they enjoyed the most. Nearly ninety percent said it was the lecture on myths. I then started giving presentations outside of class on the topic, which ultimately led to the idea of writing this book.

We are continually bombarded with information related to our health. This information comes from newspapers, television, the internet, magazines, radio, friends, and even family members (think of all the health-related advice you have received from your mother and grandmother over the years). Much of the information we hear is simply not true. Often the latest study on a given topic will create a buzz, and a new fad will be born. The fad will last for months or maybe years until subsequent studies disprove the idea.

Reading research on health-related topics can be both confusing and frustrating. Sometimes research studies do not conclusively point to one definitive answer. It's not uncommon to read research articles on a selected topic and find that different studies point to completely different conclusions. In that case, it is important to look at the complete body of work that has been done in that area (i.e., find a consensus among most of the studies). The answers to some of the questions raised in this book are very clearly supported by the research that has been conducted on that topic. However, for other topics, the answer is not so clear. In those cases, I've carefully examined the available evidence before coming to any conclusions.

Some of the information in this book may surprise you. Based upon what you believe or have heard in the past, you may even question some of what is written on the following pages. I've had people (like my wife, for instance) stand up during my talks and disagree with my findings. I really don't mind that as it keeps things interesting. I've learned that sometimes it's hard for people to accept new information or be open to ideas that are contrary to what they already believe, especially if they have had those beliefs for many years or if the original information comes from their grandmother, because for many people grandmothers are usually right!

SECTION ONE

EXERCISE and FITNESS

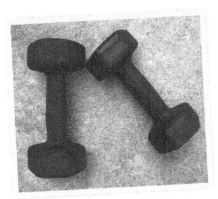

ONCE YOU STOP EXERCISING, MUSCLE CAN TURN TO FAT...

FALSE

MYTH 1

SO YOU DECIDE to take a break from your exercise routine, which regularly included a variety of cardiovascular and resistance training exercises performed three days a week. After a couple of months you notice a big change in your body composition. You start to see more fat and less muscle, so naturally you think that your muscles are already turning into fat. Well, the truth is that muscle and fat are two distinctly different types of tissue or cells (Martini and Nath 2009). Fat doesn't turn into muscle when you start exercising, just as muscle doesn't turn into fat if you stop. There are many different types of cells in the body: bone cells, skin cells, fat cells, red blood cells, etc. Since muscle and fat are different types of cells, they have different characteristics and functions and therefore react to exercise, or lack thereof, in different ways. When you start exercising, especially resistance training or weight lifting, your muscle cells can increase in size. This is

Martini, F. and Nath, J. *Fundamentals of Anatomy and Physiology*, 8th ed., pp. 125, 296. Pearson Benjamin Cummings: San Francisco, CA, 2009.

called hypertrophy. Hypertrophy usually only occurs if you work your muscles beyond the level that they are used to. If you have been exercising for some time and then stop, your muscle cells can actually decrease in size. This is called atrophy. Likewise, if you gain fat weight on your body, your fat cells simply increase in size, just as they will decrease in size if you lose fat weight. So it is possible that fat could occupy space where there was once muscle, but just as ligaments don't turn to bone and rocks don't turn to metal, muscle does not turn into fat. It is possible for your fat cells and muscle cells to both increase at the same time. This could happen if you started lifting weights and simultaneously greatly increased your caloric consumption. Sometimes people say that they don't want to start lifting weights because they are afraid that if they stop, the muscle will just turn to fat, but that is just not possible.

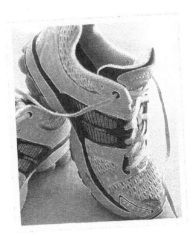

YOU WILL BURN MORE CALORIES IF YOU RUN A MILE THAN IF YOU WALK A MILE...

TRUE

THIS IS A topic that is actually discussed a fair amount by health and fitness experts. As with most topics, the research findings are somewhat varied; however, most studies show that you do burn more calories when you run than when you walk. On average, you burn about eighty calories when you walk a mile and one hundred calories when you run a mile. One study, performed by Hall, et al. (2004), examined the number of calories burned when research participants either walked a mile on a treadmill at just over three miles per hour or ran a mile on a treadmill at just over six miles per hour. In this study the walkers burned eighty-one calories and the runners burned 114 calories after covering the one mile distance. If you have ever had a physics course, you probably learned that moving a certain amount of mass a given distance will require a certain amount of energy. If you apply this principle to the question about the caloric expenditure of

Hall, C., Figueroa, A., Fernhall, B., and Kanaley, J. Energy expenditure of walking and running: Comparison with prediction equations. *Medicine and Science in Sports and Exercise* (2004), Vol 36, pp. 2128-2134.

walking vs. running, it would appear that the same number of calories should be burned whether you walk or run because you are simply moving a specific amount of mass (your body) a specific distance (a mile). Why is it, then, that the caloric requirement is higher for running? It turns out that walking is a slightly more efficient way of moving and requires fewer muscles than running. Picture your legs when you walk. They are somewhat straight, and they don't bend all that much. Also, when you walk, your center of gravity stays fairly constant, and there is minimal contact with the ground. On the other hand, when you run, your legs usually bend more; you expend more energy pushing off to propel yourself; and you actually elevate yourself in the air a bit as well. So running a mile does in fact burn more calories than walking a mile.

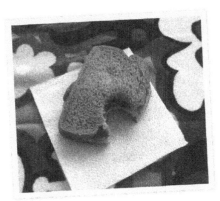

SWIMMING AFTER EATING A MEAL IS DANGEROUS...

FALSE

I'M SAD TO write that over the past two hundred years or so hundreds of thousands, maybe even millions, of idle hours have been spent by children wishing they could immediately jump or dive back into a lake, river, or pool after they had consumed a meal. These precious recreational hours were lost because the children were under the close and watchful eye of their mother or father who believed it was dangerous to swim after eating. As I fondly think back to my childhood, I recall how well-intentioned adults taught me how to swim by throwing me into a lake in water over my head, yet how my mother would not let me swim for at least an hour after having eaten a peanut butter and jelly sandwich. The idea that it is not safe to swim after eating has been around for a long time. However, as hard as I looked in the research and medical literature, I could not find one report of a drowning or near drowning due to swimming immediately after eating.

Steinhaus, A. Evidence and opinions related to swimming after meals. *Journal of Health, Physical Education, and Recreation* (1961), Vol 32, p. 59.

Anecdotally, I think that the hundreds of thousands of kids who eat and then immediately resume playing in community pools, lakes, etc. are evidence that there is little to no risk in doing so. The thought is that if you swim after you eat, blood will be diverted from your exercising muscles to your stomach to help with the digestion process, resulting in severe cramping. In an article on the topic published in 1961, however, Arthur Steinhaus claims that the body will supply the exercising muscles with the blood and oxygen needed before diverting blood to the stomach. In his article, Steinhaus also mentions how the myth may have been perpetuated by older versions of the Red Cross First Aid Instructors book, which contained recommendations about not swimming after eating and by such folklore as American Indians massaging the abdomen after meals to make swimming safe. Having a full stomach when you jump into the pool might make for an uncomfortable swim, but it is not dangerous.

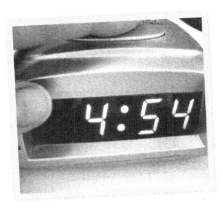

MORNING WORKOUTS ELEVATE YOUR METABOLISM MORE THAN EVENING WORKOUTS...

FALSE

MANY, DARE I say fanatical, people set their alarm clocks for 4:30 a.m. so they can get to the gym by 5:00 a.m. for an early morning workout. Some have no other choice, some actually enjoy a pre-sunrise sweat session, and some have to peel themselves out of bed, believing that a workout early in the morning results in more calories burned throughout the day. Their thinking is that exercising in the morning will elevate their metabolism to a higher level than a later work-out and that it will stay elevated during the remainder of their daily activities. On the flip side, there is also the belief that if you work out before going to bed, you'll burn fewer calories because you are not up and moving around. Both scenarios are false. The truth is that three hundred calories burned during a 5:00 a.m. workout or a 9:00 p.m. workout is simply three hundred calories burned. There has actually been a fair number of research studies done on this topic. For example, Galliven,

Galliven, E., Singh, A., Michelson, D., Bina, S., Gold, W., and Deuster, P. Hormonal and metabolic responses to exercise across time of day and menstrual cycle. *Journal of Applied Physiology* (1997), Vol 83, pp. 1822-1831.

et al. (1997) studied metabolic and hormonal responses of participants who worked out at different times of the day at high (ninety percent) or moderate (seventy percent) intensities. The authors concluded that the time of day at which the participants exercised (morning vs. evening) had no impact on the number of calories burned during the workout. One thing that is believed to be true is that many people can't exercise as hard in the morning as they can later in the day. This is thought to be due to a decreased body temperature early in the morning as well as decreased flexibility and lower levels of alertness and vigor. So if you've been struggling to get yourself out of bed at 5:00 in the morning because you think you will burn more calories in your spinning class, by all means stay in bed! The best advice anyone could ever give about scheduling your daily workout is that you should exercise at a time which is convenient and appealing to you.

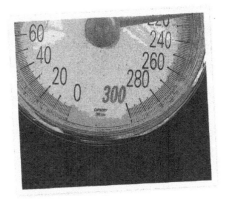

IT IS HEALTHIER TO BE 25 POUNDS OVERWEIGHT AND PHYSICALLY ACTIVE THAN TO BE AT YOUR OPTIMAL WEIGHT AND SEDENTARY...

TRUE

VERY OFTEN FITNESS and thinness go hand in hand, but thin does not automatically imply excellent health. When you see someone who is overweight or obese, do you assume that the individual is unhealthy and lazy or that he or she over-eats, doesn't work out, and is at an increased risk for disease? Likewise, when you see someone who is thin, do you usually presume that person must exercise, is fit, and is likely to be healthy? Surprisingly, a person who looks thin could actually have a high percentage of body fat, be sedentary, have poor cardiorespiratory endurance, and overall might not be all that healthy. On the other hand, current research is starting to support the idea that physical activity, even in people who are overweight or obese, has a powerful protective effect on health. This is often referred to as the "fitness vs. fatness" debate. There have been hundreds of studies performed related to obesity, exercise, and health. Regretfully, a large

Blair, S. and Brodney, S. Effects of physical inactivity and obesity on morbidity and mortality: Current research evidence and research issues. *Medicine and Science in Sports and Exercise* (1999), Vol 31, pp. S646-62.

percentage of these studies have not taken into consideration the fitness level of participants when determining risk for chronic diseases. Blair and Brodney (1999) published a review on the topic titled "Effects of Physical Inactivity and Obesity on Morbidity and Mortality: Current Evidence and Research Issues." These authors reviewed twenty-four very high-quality research studies and concluded that "overweight and obese individuals who were active and fit had morbidity and mortality rates that were at least as low, and in many instances much lower, than normal weight individuals who were sedentary." This comes as a surprise to many people, but the message is clear: whether you are overweight or not, physical activity can have a tremendous positive impact on your health and quality of life. So get out there and get moving!

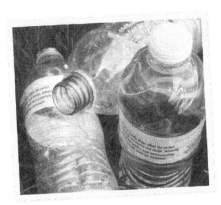

IT IS POSSIBLE TO DRINK TOO MUCH WATER WHEN EXERCISING...

TRUE

IMAGINE A PERSON you know who is in really, really good shape. Imagine that person in mile nineteen of a marathon on a hot sunny afternoon. Suddenly, he or she starts to feel fatigued and dizzy and collapses on the course—a true medical emergency. This type of scenario is fairly common and is sometimes caused by a condition called hyponatremia. In fact, Rogers and Hew-Butler (2009) state that hyponatremia can now be considered the most important medical problem of endurance exercise. Hyponatremia occurs when sodium concentrations in the body become dangerously low. Sodium and other electrolytes are important for muscle, heart, and brain function. Exercise-associated hyponatremia usually occurs when athletes are participating in long distance endurance events (e.g., marathon or ironman); they are sweating a lot and only drinking water. To understand how only drinking water can lower sodium concentrations in the body, imagine

Rogers, I. and Hew-Butler, T. Exercise-associated hyponatremia: Overzealous fluid consumption. *Wilderness and Environmental Medicine* (2009), Vol 20, pp. 139-143.

taking a glass of salt water and pouring twenty-five percent of it out. You then replace what you poured out with water; the sodium concentration of the fluid in the glass will be less than when you started. The same thing happens in our bodies, and it can be a very dangerous condition. Signs and symptoms of hyponatremia include headache, nausea, confusion, dizziness, fatigue, slurred speech, cramps, seizures, and coma, and the condition can even result in death. Luckily it is fairly easy to prevent hyponatremia. Individuals participating in long distance endurance events such as marathons should drink both water and a sports drink that contains electrolytes, or they should try to consume some food during the event that contains sodium. Happy running!

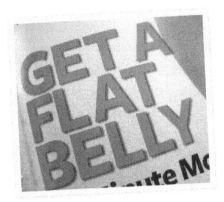

SIT-UPS
MAKE YOUR
STOMACH
FLATTER...

FALSE

HAVE YOU EVER started doing sit-ups, crunches, planks, oblique twists, reverse curls, and other abdominal exercises in the hope of getting a flatter stomach? If you have, you are not alone. Millions of people would like to flatten their tummies and improve their overall appearance. If you are like lots of other people, you quickly learned that hundreds or even thousands of crunches and sit-ups will do little to nothing to flatten your midsection and give you that coveted six-pack. A research study conducted by Katch, et al. (1984) examined whether sit-up training had any impact on abdominal fat cell size in research participants. The researchers had participants do an intensive training routine, which consisted of doing sit-ups five days a week for twenty-seven days. In total, participants performed over five thousand sit-ups. That averages out to more than 185 sit-ups a day. After the study was complete, the authors concluded, "In summary, the results of the present

Katch, F., Clarkson, P., Kroll, W., and McBride, T. Effects of sit up exercise training on adipose cell size and adiposity. *Research Quarterly for Exercise and Sport* (1984), Vol 55, pp. 242-247.

experiment have demonstrated that sit up exercise training did not preferentially reduce the diameter of abdominal adipose [fat] cells, and did not significantly alter the thickness of the abdominal subcutaneous fat layer or abdominal circumference." In short, sit-ups didn't decrease the observable fat thickness in the abdomen. Doing sit-ups and other abdominal exercises isn't a bad thing; these types of exercises can help strengthen and tone the midsection. But realize that they alone won't flatten your stomach. Losing even a few pounds of body fat will likely result in your stomach beginning to look flatter.

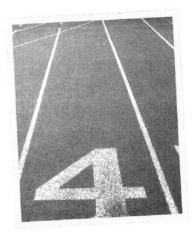

STATIC STRETCHING BEFORE SPRINTING OR JUMPING DECREASES PERFORMANCE...

TRUE

I, LIKE MANY of you reading this book, had the opportunity to participate in sports all through middle school and high school. For as long as I can remember, I have seen coaches instruct their athletes to perform static stretching prior to being active in practice or competitions. I've seen this occur at the high school level, college level, and even in professional sports. A static stretch means holding a stretch position for twenty or thirty seconds, sometimes even longer. The thinking was that static stretching prior to activity helped loosen up the muscles and improve athletic performance. However, research conducted on this topic over the past five to ten years is starting to suggest otherwise, especially for explosive type movements such as sprinting and jumping. Ian Shrier published a review article on this topic in the *Clinical Journal of Sports Medicine* (2004), and in it he examined studies that had participants perform static stretching prior to explosive

Shrier, I. Does stretching improve performance? A systematic and critical review of the literature. *Clinical Journal of Sports Medicine* (2004), Vol 14, pp. 267-273.

type activities. Dr. Shrier concluded that "In summary, the evidence suggests that stretching immediately prior to exercise decreases the results on performance tests that require isolated force or power." It should be noted that it is still recommended that static stretching be performed after exercise and that post exercise stretching has been shown to positively impact performance. If static stretching is not recommended prior to explosive type activities, then what should we do? Most fitness specialists now recommend that you complete a light cardiovascular warm-up for ten or twelve minutes prior to activity, something at an intensity level that will get your blood flowing and result in a light sweat. Experts also recommend that people perform dynamic stretches or dynamic warm-ups prior to activity. Movements that mimic those which will be required in a particular practice or event might be ideal.

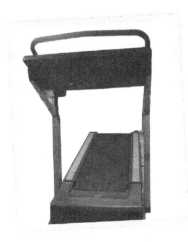

EXERCISING ON A REGULAR BASIS ADDS YEARS TO YOUR LIFE...

TRUE

DO YOU ENGAGE in physical activity on a regular basis? If you do, research is starting to show that your health, on average, is improved because of it. People have engaged in physical activity for health benefits for thousands of years, but it hasn't been until the last twenty or thirty years that we have truly realized just how beneficial getting out and strapping on our walking shoes can be. Being active on a regular basis is correlated with many health benefits. Some of those benefits include helping us maintain a healthy weight; fighting off depression; preventing heart disease, stroke, and cancer; and improving our self confidence and self esteem. I could easily fill this page with nothing but health benefits that come from being active. It shouldn't be much of a surprise, then, to learn that being active on a consistent basis adds years to your life. Research has shown that there is an inverse relationship between physical activity and mortality. That is, as one

Lee, I. and Skerrett, P. Physical activity and all-cause mortality: What is the dose-response relation? *Medicine and Science in Sports and Exercise* (2001), Vol 33, pp. S459-S471.

variable goes up (physical activity), the other (mortality) goes down. Roughly speaking, people with low to moderate levels of physical activity live one to two years longer than those who engage in no physical activity, and those with high levels of physical activity live about three to four years longer. Authors of a review article published on this topic in the journal *Medicine and Science in Sports and Exercise* (2001) stated, "We identified 44 studies conducted in Canada, Denmark, Finland, Germany, Israel, Italy, the Netherlands, Norway, Sweden, the United Kingdom, and the United States that addressed this issue. Based on these studies, there is clear evidence of an inverse dose-response relation between volume of physical activity (or level of physical fitness) and all-cause mortality. The preponderance of evidence suggests that risk of dying during a given period continues to decline with increasing levels of physical activity." So if someone tells you to take a hike, they are actually giving you good advice.

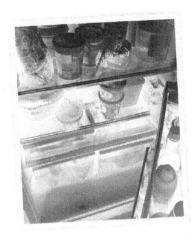

YOU EAT MORE AFTER YOU START AN EXERCISE PROGRAM...

TRUE & FALSE

MYTH 10

I SOMETIMES HEAR people say they are hungrier and eat more after they start an exercise program. I've even heard people say they are afraid to start working out because they think it will stimulate their appetite, which might lead to their gaining weight because of their increased activity level. The research on this topic is a bit mixed but leans in the direction of a person's appetite not increasing due to increased levels of activity. A review study by Martins, et al. (2008), published in the *International Journal of Obesity*, examined many of the studies conducted on this topic. The authors concluded that "There is a large body of evidence supporting a beneficial role of exercise on appetite regulation. Exercise has been shown to lead to a more sensitive eating behavior in response to previous energy intake and not to induce any acute/chronic physiological adaptations that would lead to an increase in hunger and/ or energy intake in the short term." But not so fast. It appears

Martins, C., Morgan, L., and Truby, H. A review of the effects of exercise on appetite regulation: An obesity perspective. *International Journal of Obesity* (2008), Vol 32, pp. 1337-1347.

that gender might play a role in whether we are tempted to run to the nearest buffet following a five mile jog or a swim in our local pool. Martins and colleagues did reference a number of studies that showed that energy intake (calories consumed) often increases in women following acute periods of physical activity. Now that really doesn't seem fair! Why might it be that women get hungry following exercise and men do not? It may be that the hormones responsible for helping regulate our energy intake (e.g., ghrelin, insulin, leptin) respond differently in women and men following exercise. Fair or not, this should not discourage women from engaging in physical activity. However, it would be helpful if women were aware that following exercise they might experience an increase in appetite so that they can take appropriate measures (e.g., have health snacks on hand) to quell their appetites rather than supersizing an order of french fries.

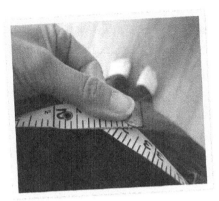

IT IS POSSIBLE TO TARGET FAT REDUCTION IN YOUR ABS, HIPS, AND THIGHS...

FALSE

AS MUCH AS most of us would like to, we simply can't start doing crunches, lunges, and leg lifts and magically burn fat from our abs, buttocks, and thighs. Generally speaking, fat is usually referred to as visceral fat (surrounding internal organs) or subcutaneous fat (under the skin). It is the subcutaneous fat we often try to impact with diet and exercise in an attempt to improve our appearance and overall health. The notion that we can target fat reduction in specific parts of the body is referred to as spot reduction. However, it is almost universally agreed upon in the medical and scientific communities that spot reduction is not possible. Metabolically speaking, fat isn't connected to the muscle it covers; in other words, when you work certain muscles you will not burn calories from the fat that covers those muscles. One of the earliest studies on this topic was conducted by Gwinup and colleagues (1971) and published in the *Annals of Internal Medicine*. These authors

Gwinup, G., Chelvam, R., and Steinberg, T. Thickness of subcutaneous fat and activity of underlying muscles. *Annals of Internal Medicine* (1971), Vol 74, pp. 408-411.

looked at fat in the arms of tennis players who had played tennis no less than six hours a week for two or more years. The researchers reported that the tennis players had increased muscle mass in the arm they played tennis with (which was to be expected), but found no reduction in the fat in that arm. The authors concluded that "The significant finding in this study is that the greater amount of exercise in the playing arm of tennis players is not accompanied by diminished fat deposits over the arm." As we exercise and burn fat, we burn fat from all parts of our bodies, not isolated locations. It can be frustrating when you are working hard to lose inches in certain areas of your body and you are not seeing the results you would like. The best advice I can give is to stay positive, be consistent with your activity regimen, and focus on healthy eating habits. You will eventually see the results you are looking for!

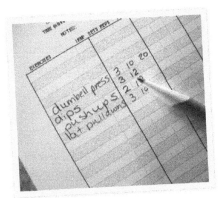

THE SORENESS YOU FEEL AFTER EXERCISING IS CAUSED BY LACTIC ACID BUILDUP...

FALSE

MOST PEOPLE HAVE experienced delayed onset muscle soreness (DOMS). If you have ever gone from living a relatively sedentary lifestyle to starting an exercise program and possibly overdoing it on the first day, you have likely experienced severe soreness! DOMS is the pain and stiffness that is felt twelve to twenty-four hours after exercise. It can last for up to seventy-two hours but often resolves within forty-eight hours of your workout. The pain and discomfort experienced from DOMS can range from mild to severe. Some people don't mind DOMS that is mild in nature as it serves as a reminder that they have been working their muscles. However, most people don't like severe DOMS that limits mobility and function and results in severe pain. Eccentric muscle contractions, which occur when muscles are loaded in a lengthened position, usually result in increased levels of DOMS. Downhill running, the lowering phase of a biceps curl, and the downward motion

Wilmore, J. and Costill, D. *Physiology of Sport and Exercise*, 3rd ed., Human Kinetics: Champaign, IL, 2004.

of a squat are examples of eccentric muscle actions. Many people mistakenly believe that DOMS is caused by lactic acid buildup in the muscles, but that is not true. It is true that lactic acid can accumulate in working muscles; however, lactic acid is usually no longer present in muscles forty-five to sixty minutes following a workout. In a very well-respected exercise physiology textbook, Wilmore and Costill (2004) state, "We now are confident that muscle soreness results from injury or damage to the muscle itself, generally the muscle fiber and possibly the sarcolemma." Keep in mind that this "injury" the authors are referring to is many very small tears that occur in the muscle at a microscopic level. The best way to prevent DOMS is to avoid it all together. This usually can be accomplished by gently easing into an exercise regimen and slowly increasing the duration and intensity of your workouts.

NUTRITION

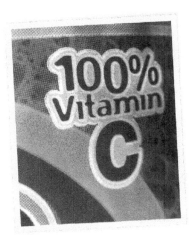

VITAMIN C HELPS PREVENT COLDS...

FALSE

IF YOU ARE one of the millions who rush to the store for vitamin C at the first sign of the sniffles, current research findings suggest that you may be wasting your money. For many years the question of whether vitamin C can prevent colds has been controversial. Vitamin C was the very first vitamin to be isolated and was artificially synthesized in the 1930's; however, it wasn't until the 1970's that the topic generated great public interest when Linus Pauling (awarded Nobel Prizes in chemistry and peace) widely publicized previous research results suggesting that vitamin C might help prevent colds. Over the next decade a large number of well-designed studies were conducted to try and replicate this earlier research. Many of these studies have been summarized in a review article published by Hemila, et al. (2009), which only considered studies in which participants received two hundred milligrams or more of vitamin C per day and also used placebo comparisons (an

Hemila, H., Chalker, E., Treacy, B., and Douglas, B. Vitamin C for preventing and treating the common cold. *Cochrane Database Systematic Reviews* (2009), Issue 3, CD000980.

indicator of a higher quality study). The results of thirty studies, which together had over eleven thousand research participants, revealed that vitamin C had little effect on whether they caught a cold or not. The authors concluded, "The failure of vitamin C supplementation to reduce the incidence of colds in the normal population indicates that routine megadose prophylaxis is not rationally justified for community use." For most people, vitamin C supplementation doesn't help prevent colds. Interestingly, six studies in which marathon runners and skiers were exposed to periods of extreme physical or cold stress showed that vitamin C supplementation did cut the risk of developing a cold by fifty percent. So if you engage in physically demanding activities, especially in cold weather, vitamin C might help you fend off a cold.

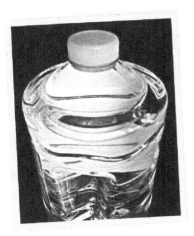

IT IS IMPORTANT TO DRINK AT LEAST 64 OUNCES OF WATER A DAY...

FALSE

MANY PEOPLE BELIEVE that most of us are walking around in a chronic state of dehydration. That really is not true. It is hard to read an article written about health and not see the recommendation to drink at least sixty-four ounces of water a day, simply referred to as 8 X 8 (eight glasses of water each holding eight ounces), and many are heeding this advice. The next time you're out in public, pay attention to what people are carrying—water bottles seem to have become a nationwide trend. They often reflect the owner's personality, adorned with logos and colorful designs. Some are indestructible, and many are being made from aluminum or other metals. I even see a few workout fanatics at the gym who carry plastic gallon milk jugs filled with water to stay properly hydrated. It is important that we consume enough water (our bodies are sixty to seventy percent water) because we lose water when we breathe, sweat, urinate, and have bowel

Valtin, H. "Drink at least eight glasses of water a day." Really? Is there scientific evidence for "8 X 8"? *The American Journal of Physiology – Regulatory, Integrative and Comparative Physiology* (2002), Vol 283, pp. 993-1004.

movements; and our water loss can be even greater when we are sick, pregnant, or spending time in high altitude. How much water we lose can be influenced by our age, health, activity level, and the climate we live in. Generally speaking, we should replace the amount of water lost from our bodies on a daily basis. Most of us do this via the foods we consume (fifteen to twenty-five percent of our fluid intake is from food) and by drinking when we are thirsty. The Institute of Medicine recommends consuming seventy to one hundred ounces of fluids a day, from sources such as food, milk, water, juice, tea, coffee, etc. In one of the few published articles I could find on this topic Heinz Valtin (2002) states, "Despite an extensive search of the literature and many personal inquiries and discussions with nutritionists and colleagues, I have found no scientific reports concluding that we all must drink at least eight glasses of water a day."

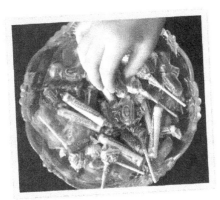

EATING SUGAR MAKES KIDS HYPERACTIVE...

FALSE

IF YOU ARE a parent and have ever had the honor of hosting a birthday party for your child, I can understand how you might think that sugar (e.g., cake, soda, candy, cookies) immediately enters the bloodstream and is magically converted to pure energy (jet fuel?) resulting in superhuman-like bursts of activity in your kids. The research studies on this topic, however, tell a different story. In an article published in the journal *Critical Reviews in Food Science and Nutrition*, Krummel, et al. (1996) state, "Twelve double-blind, placebo-controlled studies of sugar challenges failed to provide any evidence that sugar ingestion leads to untoward behavior in children with Attention-Deficit Hyperactivity Disorder or in normal children." In other words, when children consume sugar, it does not result in increased activity levels. In fact, the results of some of the studies suggest that sugar might result in a calming effect for some children. Why then do so many people

Krummel, D., Seligson, F., and Guthrie, H. Hyperactivity: Is candy causal? *Critical Reviews in Food Science and Nutrition* (1996), Vol 36, pp. 31-47.

believe that sugar causes kids to be hyper? It is understandable how some would associate things like cake, cookies, candy, and ice cream at parties with increased activity levels in children. Anecdotally, this has been happening for many years with both parents and teachers. Might it just be that kids are more excited and active at a birthday party because they have ten of their best friends to play with? My wife and I have hosted our fair share of birthday parties (we have three boys), and I can honestly say that I've tried to pay attention to the activity level of the kids attending the parties before as well as after the cake and ice cream have been served, the result being no noticeable difference. We even engage in the questionable practice of letting our kids eat lots of candy right after they are done trick or treating. But when we put them to bed, they quickly fall asleep just like they do every other night.

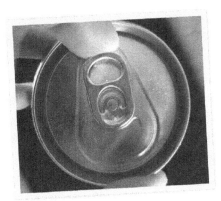

DRINKING BEER IN MODERATION IS GOOD FOR YOUR HEALTH...

TRUE

IT MIGHT SEEM too good to be true, but drinking beer in moderation is good for your health. It is widely known and almost universally accepted that drinking red wine is good for your heart, but research is now showing that the same health benefits hold true for consuming beer and hard liquor in moderation. The "in moderation" is really the key. Moderation for women is usually defined as one drink per day and one to two drinks per day for men. College students in my courses often ask if it is all right to abstain from drinking for five days and then have eight or ten drinks on a Friday night. Sorry, but that is not moderation. It also should be noted that consuming alcohol in excess increases the risk for cardiovascular disease. So how much alcohol actually constitutes a serving or a drink? For beer it is twelve ounces, five ounces for wine, and 1.5 ounces for hard liquor. The first indication that alcohol might have a protective effect on the heart came in the early 1900's

Klatsky, A. Drink to your health? *Scientific American Special Edition* (2006), Vol 16, pp. 22-29.

when those performing autopsies on people who died of cirrhosis of the liver found that arteries in these same individuals showed little to no sign of atherosclerosis (the fatty deposits on the inside of the artery walls). At first it was thought that alcohol may have acted like a solvent dissolving this unwanted and unhealthy fat. Most studies done on this topic show that consuming alcohol in moderation results in a twenty to thirty percent decrease in risk for cardiovascular disease (Klatsky 2006). So the question is why? Current thinking is that alcohol helps elevate HDL or good cholesterol (HDL levels in moderate drinkers are ten to twenty percent higher than non drinkers) and also decreases blood clotting capacity in the body. Increased levels of HDL could help guard against atherosclerosis, and decreased clotting capacity (when platelets are less sticky) could decrease the risk of having a heart attack.

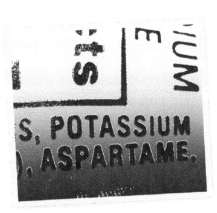

ASPARTAME HAS BEEN SHOWN TO CAUSE LUPUS, MULTIPLE SCLEROSIS, AND CANCER...

FALSE

MILLIONS OF PEOPLE enjoy sweetening their coffee, tea, cereal, etc. with aspartame, and/or they consume products such as diet soda that contain aspartame. Aspartame is usually added to products such as Nutrasweet, or you may also see it as a sugar substitute called Equal. There is no question that aspartame is widely consumed; some of the reasons might be that it is very sweet (roughly 180 times sweeter than sugar) and that it contains few calories. Aspartame was accidently discovered in the mid 1960's by an individual who was working on a drug to prevent ulcers. It was approved for human consumption by the Food and Drug Administration in the early 1980's. Of all the health myths and misconceptions that I've written and spoken about, the safety of aspartame certainly is one of the most contentious. Many people believe that consuming aspartame can increase an individual's risk

Butchko, H., Stargel, W., Comer, P., Mayhew, D., Benninger, C., Blackburn, G., De Sonneville, L., Geha, R., Hertelendy, Z., Koestner, A., Leon, A., Liepa, G., McMartin, K., Mendenhall, C., Munro, I., Novotny, E., Renwick, A., Schiffman, S., Schomer, D., and Shaywitz, B. Aspartame: Review of safety. *Regulatory Toxicology and Pharmacology* (2002), Vol 35, pp. S1-S93.

for cancer, seizures, multiple sclerosis, lupus, and a variety of other diseases and conditions. I recently keyed in "aspartame" on an internet search engine and came up with nearly two million hits. It wasn't uncommon to come across statements such as "Aspartame is, by far, the most dangerous substance on the market that is added to foods." However, aspartame has been widely researched as well. In a large review article published in the journal *Regulatory Toxicology and Pharmacology* (2002) examining many studies that have been done on aspartame, Harriett Butchko and colleagues state, "When all the research on aspartame, including evaluations in both the premarketing and postmarketing periods, is examined as a whole, it is clear that aspartame is safe, and there are no unresolved questions regarding its safety under conditions of intended use."

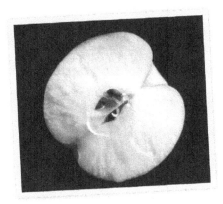

THERE IS A SMALL AMOUNT OF CAFFEINE IN AN APPLE...

FALSE

ONE DAY AS I was giving a lecture in my college level health and wellness course, a student asked a question which I had to admit that I couldn't answer. The student had asked, "Is it true that there is caffeine in an apple"? My initial response was "I don't think so," but I had to be honest and tell the class that I wasn't completely sure. I had been through eleven years of college courses and had been teaching health and wellness classes at the college level for nearly ten years, and I had never heard anything about there being caffeine in apples. As I continued to teach that particular lecture, the student's question kept popping into my mind. I remember thinking, "If there really is caffeine in apples, how could I not know about it!" I decided to ask the rest of the class if they had ever heard that there was caffeine in apples. To my surprise, nearly twenty percent of the class raised their hands. One enthusiastic student even said that her mother had recently told her that there

Sizer, F. and Whitney, E. *Nutrition Concepts and Controversies*, 11th ed., pp. A-16, Thomson Wadsworth: Belmont, CA, 2008.

was more caffeine in an apple than in a regular cup of coffee. I could hardly wait for class to finish and get back into my office to find out what the answer to the student's question really was. Once in my office I did a quick internet search and realized that this is a fairly common misconception. There is no caffeine in apples. So why do some people think there is? I've heard people say that they feel like they have more energy after they eat an apple. This certainly may be true, but it's not due to caffeine. A raw medium-sized apple contains carbohydrates, fiber, iron, potassium, zinc, vitamin A, and vitamin C, (Sizer and Whitney 2008). Also, there is caffeic acid in apples (caffeic acid is a phenol found in fruits and vegetables that has antioxidant properties); some might confuse this with caffeine. So an apple a day might help keep the doctor away, but not because there is caffeine in it.

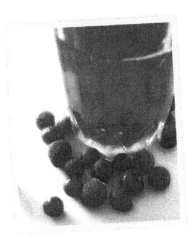

DRINKING CRANBERRY JUICE IS AN EFFECTIVE TREATMENT FOR URINARY TRACT INFECTIONS...

FALSE

IT APPEARS THAT over the past ten to fifteen years cranberries have experienced an explosion in popularity. A quick internet search revealed that cranberry juice is being combined with a number of other juices (e.g., apple, grape, pomegranate), and cranberries can be found in a wide variety of products such as tea, coffee, salsa, butter, soap, fudge, cookies, pancake mix, mustard (yes, mustard!), trail mix, syrup, jam, muffins, and even BBQ sauce. One potential reason for this increase in popularity might be the common belief that cranberries can be used to effectively treat urinary tract infections (UTI). A UTI results when the amount of bacteria in the urine reaches a certain level or threshold. The primary culprit responsible for the majority of UTI's is the E coli bacteria. There are millions of cases of UTI's reported annually to hospitals and clinics, and they are usually experienced more frequently in women than men. It was once thought that drinking cranberry juice increased the acidity of the urine, thus killing the

Jepson, R., Mihaljevic, L., and Craig, J. Cranberries for treating urinary tract infections. *Cochrane Database of Systematic Reviews* (1998), Issue 4, Art. No. CD001322. DOI: 10.1002/14651858.CD001322.

bacteria that were causing a UTI. However, this is no longer believed to be true. There is some evidence that substances in cranberries might decrease the ability of bacteria to attach to the inner lining of the bladder, thus potentially decreasing the incidence of UTI's. However, there is little to no research supporting the use of cranberry juice to treat urinary tract infections. Jepson and colleagues (1998) reviewed the research in this area and concluded that "No randomized controlled trials have been performed to assess the effectiveness of cranberry juice or cranberry products for the treatment of UTI's. Therefore, at the present time, there is no evidence to suggest that cranberry juice or other cranberry products are effective in treating UTI's."

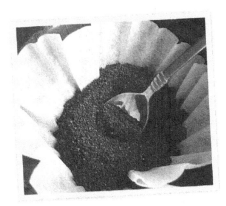

COFFEE AND OTHER CAFFEINATED BEVERAGES CAUSE DEHYDRATION...

FALSE

CAFFEINE IS ONE of the most widely consumed substances known to man—I say that as I sit writing this and sipping my morning coffee. It is true that caffeine is a diuretic, meaning that it will cause the kidneys to excrete more urine. Research dating back to the 1920's has shown this. However, consuming caffeine will not result in dehydration. Dehydration is defined as excessive loss of body water. Symptoms often include muscle spasms and cramping, headaches, fatigue, dizziness, and decreased performance. These symptoms usually become noticeable only after losing about two percent of the total water volume you have in your body. It is such a widespread belief that caffeine causes dehydration that even some healthcare providers tell this to their patients. Someone recently shared with me that they were encouraged by their physician during a routine check-up to cut out coffee to prevent dehydration. Some doctors even tell patients to drink one glass of water for

Armstrong, L., Casa, D., Maresh, C., and Gania, M. Caffeine, fluid-electrolyte balance, temperature regulation, and exercise heat tolerance. *Exercise and Sports Sciences Reviews* (2007), Vol 35, pp. 135-140.

every cup of coffee or other caffeinated beverage consumed. The truth is that the diuretic effect of caffeine is too mild to cause dehydration. For example, if you were to consume fifty ounces of coffee, you may lose five ounces of fluid due to the diuretic effect of the caffeine, but you would still be at a positive net gain of forty-five ounces of fluid. Lawrence Armstrong and colleagues (2007) state in an article published in the journal *Exercise and Sport Sciences Reviews* that "there is no evidence to suggest that moderate caffeine intake induces chronic dehydration or negatively affects exercise performance, temperature regulation, and circulatory strain in a hot environment. Caffeinated fluids contribute to the daily human water requirements in a manner that is similar to pure water." So have that morning cup without fear of dehydration.

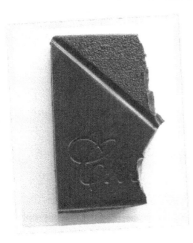

EATING CHOCOLATE, POTATO CHIPS, AND OTHER OILY AND GREASY FOODS MAKES ACNE WORSE...

FALSE

I WAS PLAGUED by pretty severe acne during my early to mid teenage years. Like millions of other people with acne, I dealt as best I could with the embarrassment that came with frequent skin outbreaks and the mild scarring sometimes left behind. I vividly remember being told by relatives, my friends' parents, and even teachers to avoid oily and greasy foods as consuming things like pizza, chocolate, hamburgers, french fries, potato chips, ice cream, and cookies could cause acne or result in an existing outbreak getting worse. If oily and greasy foods are not responsible for acne, then what is? Most experts agree that hormones play a major role and are one of the primary causes of acne. This could explain why acne often affects people from about the age of twelve into the early twenties as these are the years when hormone levels tend to fluctuate greatly. Stress is also thought to play a contributing role in acne. With stress often come changes in certain hormone

Fulton, J., Plewig, G., and Kilgman, A. Effect of chocolate on acne vulgaris. *Journal of the American Medical Association* (1969), Vol 210, pp. 2071-2074.

levels in the body, contributing to the formation of acne. Pores in the skin contain glands that make sebum (oil that lubricates skin and hair). Hormones can cause these glands to produce excessive amounts of sebum, which can then contribute to clogged pores, a buildup of bacteria, and redness and swelling (the start of acne). There has been a fair amount of research examining the impact of diet on acne. One early and often-cited study was conducted by Fulton and colleagues (1969) and published in the *Journal of the American Medical Association*. These researchers had participants consume a 112-gram chocolate bar or a control bar with no chocolate every day over a four week period and monitored acne outbreaks. When the study was completed, the authors concluded "ingestion of high amounts of chocolate did not materially affect the course of acne vulgaris or the output or composition of sebum."

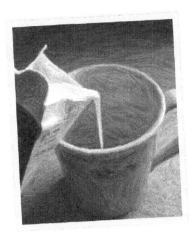

DRINKING A WARM GLASS OF MILK BEFORE BED HELPS YOU FALL ASLEEP FASTER...

FALSE

ONE EVENING WHEN I was having trouble falling asleep, I warmed up a glass of milk, feeling confident that what my mother had told me would help me fall asleep faster was true. As I started to drink the milk, I was surprised by how heating it up had, in my opinion, changed both the texture and flavor of the milk in a way I didn't particularly enjoy. Fighting through a mild feeling of nausea, I finished the milk and expected my eyelids to immediately become droopy. That didn't happen. In fact, I think that drinking the milk actually hindered my attempt to fall asleep. Many people believe that warm milk can serve as a sleeping aid; however, this belief is not supported by research. I could find no studies that showed drinking warm milk before bed decreased the time it took to fall asleep. I did find many internet sites that talked about how warm milk can help you fall asleep faster and even found a nursing standard of practice protocol for sleep disturbances

Foreman, M. and Wykle, M. Nursing standard-of-practice: Sleep disturbances in elderly patients. *Geriatric Nursing* (1995), Vol 16, pp. 238-243.

(1995) that encouraged the use of warm milk before bed, but none cited scientific references. There are several theories related to the "how" and "why" milk might make you drowsy. The first is that milk contains the hormone melatonin and the amino acid tryptophan, both believed to promote relaxation and possibly induce sleep. However, the amount of both substances in milk is very small and likely would not impact sleep. Another theory is that it is the warmth. Warmth tends to promote feelings of comfort and relaxation. I know a lot of people who drink warm tea before bed because it helps them relax. Some propose that warm milk might even take us back to when we were breast fed; after all babies often fall asleep after breastfeeding. Either way, there is no research supporting the idea that drinking warm milk will help you fall asleep faster.

EATING FIVE OR SIX SMALLER MEALS DURING THE DAY WILL INCREASE YOUR METABOLISM AND HELP YOU LOSE WEIGHT...

FALSE

Breakfast: 1 apple
1/2 C. tomato juice
1 cup of tea with honey
2 poached eggs

Meal #2: 1 orange
2 oz. baked chicken
A small piece bread
Raw carrots

Meal #3: Same as Meal # 2

Meal #4: Same as Meal #2 w

YEARS AGO WHEN I first started teaching college health courses, I taught that eating five or six smaller meals during the day elevated metabolism and helped people control their weight. The reason I taught it was that I had heard it so often in the popular fitness and nutrition press that I thought it had to be true. This idea has been debated since the 1950's when early studies suggested that individuals who ate fewer meals had more body fat. Many of these early studies were flawed in that researchers relied on participants' self-reporting their caloric consumption. Subsequent studies have shown that research subjects often underreport food intake by twenty to fifty percent, so the validity of some of those early studies is in question. More recent studies, with much better methodological design, have been conducted to actually measure the number of calories we burn based upon the number of meals we consume. In an article entitled "Impact of the Daily Meal Pattern

Bellisle, F. Impact of the daily meal pattern on energy balance. *Scandinavian Journal of Nutrition* (2004), 48, pp. 114-118.

on Energy Balance," which was published in the *Scandinavian Journal of Nutrition* (2004), France Bellisle states, "In addition, no difference in total energy expenditure has been documented as a function of daily meal number. Weight loss is not facilitated by high meal frequency." The thermal effect of feeding, the number of calories our bodies burn breaking down and absorbing the food we eat, is the same if we eat our daily calories in two meals or six meals. Eating more frequent meals throughout the day does not elevate our metabolism. Some studies show that individuals who eat more frequently during the day have higher obesity rates than those who eat less frequently. Weight loss or weight gain is really dependent upon the number of calories you take in versus the number of calories you expend. If you consume more calories than you burn, you will gain weight, and if you burn more calories than you consume, you will lose weight. The number of meals you eat per day does not impact metabolism.

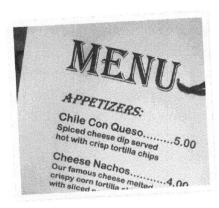

EATING AT HOME IS SAFER THAN EATING OUT...

FALSE

THE CHRISTMAS HOLIDAY party was actually a wonderful time. About a dozen graduate students and professors from my department got together to celebrate the end of a long semester. Of course it was pot luck, so everyone brought a dish or two to pass. The food was all very good, there was lots of it, and I ate far too much! I left the party at about 9:00 p.m. and said goodbye to my wife, a nurse, who had to work third shift that night. I took our three dogs for a quick walk, and then it was off to bed. I knew something was seriously wrong when I woke up at about 2:00 that morning. For the next five hours I experienced frequent and repeated bouts of violent vomiting. When my wife arrived home that morning at about 8:00, she took me to the emergency room, where a nurse gave me a shot of some anti-nausea medication to try and make me feel better. At that point I felt so bad I broke down and started to cry! I can't remember a time when I have

Surak, J. A recipe for safe food: ISO 22000 and HACCP. *Quality Progress* (2007), Vol 40, p. 25.

ever felt so horrible. The episode was likely caused by a food-related illness. The Center of Disease Control and Prevention estimates that about 76 million Americans get sick from food-related illnesses each year. Many people believe that you are more likely to get sick eating out versus eating at home. That appears not to be the case. In an article about food safety in the home, John Surak (2007) states, "Most consumers believe the primary cause of food-borne illness is unsafe food handling practices in food processing plants or restaurants. In contrast, most food safety experts believe the biggest source of food borne illness is unsafe food handling practices in the home." One reason for this misperception might be that large food recalls (think spinach, beef, and eggs) and news reports of restaurant goers becoming ill tend to get major media attention. A food-borne illness acquired in the home, on the other hand, is not usually considered newsworthy.

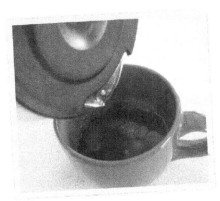

DRINKING COFFEE WILL SOBER YOU UP MORE QUICKLY AFTER A NIGHT OF DRINKING...

FALSE

IF YOU HAVE ever over-indulged and consumed too much alcohol, you probably regretted it the following day. Many party goers have awakened the day after a night of heavy drinking wishing there were some way they could expedite the "sobering up" process. Most experts agree that the only thing that will sober you up after drinking too much is time. A cold shower won't do it, a half gallon of orange juice won't do it, aspirin won't do it, and neither will black coffee. Coffee, or the caffeine in coffee, may counteract the depressive effects of alcohol, but that does not mean you are any less intoxicated. Coffee, tea, and other caffeinated beverages do nothing to lower blood alcohol content. A recent study on mice conducted at Temple University (Gulick and Gould 2009) suggests that consuming caffeine could make it more difficult to understand when you are intoxicated (especially if you're a mouse). In the study, intoxicated mice that were given caffeine

Gulick, D. and Gould, T. Effects of ethanol and caffeine on behavior in C57BL/6 mice in the plus-maze discriminative avoidance task. *Behavioral Neuroscience* (2009), Vol 123, pp. 1-8.

were more alert, but the caffeine didn't influence the mice's ability to correct learning problems or avoid things they had previously learned were harmful. When talking about what this research might mean for humans, Dr. Thomas Gould said:

> *The myth about coffee's sobering powers is particularly important to debunk because the co-use of caffeine and alcohol could actually lead to poor decisions with disastrous outcomes. People who feel tired and intoxicated after consuming alcohol may be more likely to acknowledge they are drunk. Conversely, people who have consumed both alcohol and caffeine may feel awake and competent enough to handle potentially harmful situations, such as driving while intoxicated or placing themselves in dangerous social situations.*

Remember, moderation is the key when consuming alcohol. Drunkenness can only be resolved with time, not Starbuck's.

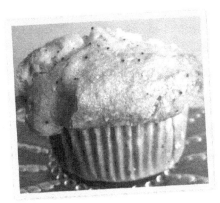

EATING A POPPY SEED MUFFIN COULD CAUSE YOU TO FAIL A DRUG TEST...

TRUE

WHAT EXACTLY IS a poppy anyway? A poppy is a colorful flower often grown in decorative gardens. However, some poppy seeds are used for food and medicine, and some are used for drugs. Many workers are required to take scheduled or unannounced drug tests at their place of employment. Drug screenings currently occur in prisons, police and fire departments, governmental agencies, the military, athletic organizations, and even in schools and private corporations. Imagine your surprise at testing positive for opiates in your blood even though you had not consumed or ingested any illicit drugs in the days, weeks, or months leading up to a drug test at work. Surprisingly, this is a fairly common occurrence. Trace amounts of opiates (morphine and codeine) can be detected in urine samples after the consumption of poppy seed bagels, muffins, or cakes. There are many documented cases of workers testing positive for opiates on drug

Meadway, C., George, S., and Braithwaite, R. Opiate concentrations following the ingestion of poppy seed products—evidence for 'the poppy seed defense'. *Forensic Science International* (1998), Vol 96, pp. 29-38.

tests and of those results being overturned after the results were challenged in court. The amount of opiates detected in a blood test after eating poppy seeds could depend on where the poppy seed was from, the type of poppy seed (there are many), weight and age of the individual consuming the poppy, and certainly how much was ingested. Currently, most of the people who test borderline positive to opiates in their systems have the results of the test reversed after follow-up testing. I even came across an article entitled "Opiate Concentrations Following the Ingestion of Poppy Seed Products—Evidence for 'the Poppy Seed Defense'," which was published in *Forensic Science International*. The authors discussed how their findings demonstrated that the poppy seed defense (e.g., claiming a positive drug test was due to poppy seed ingestion) could be used as an argument in medical, legal, and work-related cases.

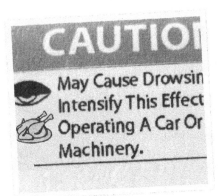

EATING TURKEY MAKES YOU DROWSY...

FALSE

YOU SLOWLY PUSH yourself away from the table after having just completed your third heaping plate of Thanksgiving dinner. The meal included mashed potatoes, gravy, stuffing, cranberry sauce, three bean salad, homemade bread, pumpkin pie, ice cream, wine, and of course lots of turkey. You slosh your way over to the sofa where you settle in and get comfortable. Your intention is to watch some Thanksgiving Day football. However, even with nearly a dozen kids running crazy through the house rambunctiously reenacting scenes from *Star Wars*, you drift off to sleep in a matter of minutes. An hour and fifteen minutes later, after getting struck by a misguided light saber strike, you wake up and realize you missed the entire fourth quarter of the game. Of course the blame for drifting off into the dream state is immediately directed at the turkey, which we all know is laced with that evil substance tryptophan. Tryptophan is an amino acid and is a precursor

Charney, D., Heninger, G., Reinhard, J., Sternberg, D., and Hafstead, K. The effect of intravenous L-tryptophan on prolactin and growth hormone and mood in healthy subjects. *Psychopharmacology* (1982), Vol 77, pp. 217-222.

(helps make) serotonin. Serotonin can be converted or turned into melatonin, which has been shown to cause sleepiness and drowsiness in humans. Research has shown that giving humans L-tryptophan can increase feelings of drowsiness (Charney, et al. 1982). However, it is widely believed that tryptophan doesn't act on the brain unless it is consumed on an empty stomach and there is no protein present in the gut (there is lots of protein in turkey). Additionally, there is not enough tryptophan in turkey to cause you to become sleepy. There is also tryptophan in eggs, beans, cheese, beef, pork, lamb, chicken, milk, barley, brown rice, fish, and peanuts, yet none of these foods are credited, or blamed, for inducing sleep. Instead, experts agree, one of the main reasons we become sleepy after we eat a big meal is that blood is diverted from the brain and other parts of the body to the stomach to aid with digestion.

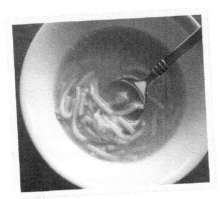

EATING CHICKEN SOUP IS HELPFUL IN TREATING THE COMMON COLD...

TRUE

AS I SIT down to write this chapter I am looking out the window at ten inches of fresh snow that was carried in by a fairly severe winter storm last night. Over the past day or so I've been exhibiting the signs and symptoms (e.g., mild coughing, scratchy throat, sniffles, a bit of nasal congestion) that would indicate I'm coming down with a cold. Impeccable timing, seeing how I've just finished researching whether or not chicken soup is helpful in treating the common cold. It is often reported that as early as the twelfth century, a physician named Moses Maimonides prescribed chicken soup for individuals suffering from asthma and upper respiratory tract ailments. Since that time, many grandmothers have continued to tout the healing powers of chicken soup. It is such a common occurrence in the Jewish tradition that chicken soup is sometimes referred to as Jewish Penicillin. Surprisingly, a fair number of research studies have been conducted on chicken

Rennard, B., Ertl, R., Gossman, G., Robbins, R., and Rennard, S. Chicken soup inhibits neutrophil chemotaxis in vitro. *Chest* (2000), Vol 118, pp. 1150-1157.

soup. In fact, these studies include examining the possible healing effects of chicken soup on pneumonia, back pain, facial pain, and even impotence (we'll save the results of those studies for another chapter). Research does show that chicken soup is beneficial for treating colds. It might be the warmth and steam that makes breathing easier and helps with congestion; it might be the fluid or ingredients like pepper, garlic, or vegetables added to the soup. Rennard and colleagues (2000), in an article published in the journal *Chest*, state that chicken soup might have an anti-inflammatory activity, namely the inhibition of neutrophil migration, and it might contain a number of substances with beneficial medicinal activity. So the next time you feel a case of the sniffles coming on, heat up a can of chicken soup.

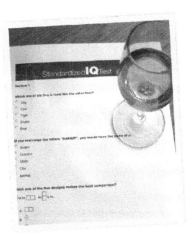

DRINKING ALCOHOL KILLS BRAIN CELLS...

FALSE

WE'VE ALL LIKELY seen a few individuals who have over-indulged and had far too much to drink. When you observe someone in that state (impaired coordination, slurred speech, uncharacteristic behaviors) and then also see what happens the following day (severe headache, dehydration, fatigue, nausea) it's easy to understand why so many people believe that drinking alcohol kills brain cells. When I was younger, I heard people (usually adults) say that getting drunk could result in the death of hundreds of thousands or even millions of brain cells. It is interesting to note here that it is estimated that the average person has over 100 billion brain cells, and we each lose roughly 200,000 brain cells a day. Contrary to what many of us have heard, drinking alcohol does not kill brain cells. A study was done in 1993 (Jensen and Pakkenberg) in which the researchers examined the number of brain cells in alcoholics and nonalcoholics who had passed away. The results

Jensen, G. and Pakkenberg, B. Do alcoholics drink their neurons away? *Lancet* (1993), Vol 342, pp. 1201.

showed no significant difference in neuron density (brain cells) between the two groups. It would be impossible to drink enough alcohol to get blood alcohol content to the level it would need to be to start killing brain cells. However, drinking can impair the cells' ability to communicate with each other. It is believed that drinking alcohol in excess can damage dendrites (the ends of nerve cells). It is also believed that, if someone stops drinking, this damage can be reversed. A large amount of research evidence is now starting to show that moderate drinking (defined as one drink per day for females and one or two drinks a day for males) can be beneficial by providing a protective effect from cognitive impairment and decreasing the risk of dementia and Alzheimer's disease.

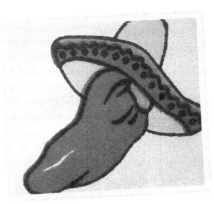

SPICY FOODS CAUSE HEARTBURN...

FALSE

A FEW YEARS ago I was at a social gathering at which there was a variety of hot and spicy foods available. I've never been one who enjoys foods that make my eyes water and give me a runny nose, but for some reason seeing others indulge in jalapeno peppers and extra hot chicken wings made me feel inadequate. That experience propelled me to start a journey, a training program of sorts, to build up my tolerance for hot and spicy foods. My training started by replacing the mild salsa in our refrigerator with the medium variety and eating a few pickled jalapenos I got from my neighbor. As I battled through the uncomfortable burning and sometime painful sensations on my tongue and in my mouth, I fully expected my venture into the world of fiery foods to result in intense heartburn, but, surprisingly, it didn't. Heartburn is the painful burning sensation felt behind the breast bone. Chronic heartburn is called gastroesophageal reflux disease (GERD).

Kaltenbach, T., Crockett, S., and Gerson, L. Are lifestyle measures effective in patients with gastroesophageal reflux disease? An evidence-based approach. *Archives of Internal Medicine* (2006), Vol 166, pp. 965-971.

The cause is related to stomach acid flowing back up the esophagus resulting in irritation and discomfort. There are many supposed contributors to GERD. Some of them include consuming things like chocolate, mint, and alcohol as well as eating beyond the point of being full, taking certain medications, sleeping in a particular body position, and smoking. Many people also believe that eating spicy food contributes to heartburn, but research suggests that this might not be the case. Authors of an article published in the journal *Archives of Internal Medicine* (2006) reviewed most of the previous studies done on GERD and stated that there was little research evidence to suggest that spicy foods contributes to GERD or that eliminating spicy foods from the diet decreases GERD symptoms. However, the authors did conclude that losing weight and elevating the head and upper back while sleeping were effective lifestyle interventions for reducing GERD.

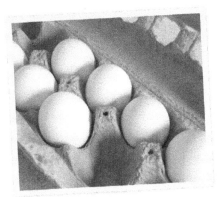

BREAKFAST SHOULD BE THE LARGEST MEAL OF THE DAY SO YOU CAN BURN OFF ALL THOSE CALORIES...

FALSE

THIS IS ANOTHER one of those myths that sounds logical even after you think about it for awhile. Eat your largest meal in the morning, and all those calories will be "burned" off as you go about your daily business. However, it is not true. Our bodies burn calories while breaking down and absorbing the food we eat. This is called diet-induced energy expenditure and is responsible for about ten percent of the calories we burn every day. This idea of making breakfast your largest meal has been around for some time and is still popular today. You've likely heard the saying "Eat breakfast like a king, lunch like a prince, and dinner like a pauper." Well, not everyone likes eating breakfast, especially a huge breakfast. This eating pattern is sometimes referred to as the reverse diet because, for most people, dinner is their largest meal of the day. I could find no scientific evidence that showed the number of calories we use to digest and store food is any different for food eaten early

Taylor, M. and Garrow, J. Compared with nibbling, neither gorging nor a morning fast affect short-term energy balance in obese patients in a chamber calorimeter. *International Journal of Obesity* (2001), Vol 25, pp. 519-528.

in the morning, during the middle of the day, or late at night. Actually, Taylor and Garrow (2001) reported that neither the number of meals we eat during the day nor a morning fast had an impact on energy expenditure. Research does show that skipping breakfast and consuming more calories later in the day is related to obesity. However, there is not a cause and effect relationship between these two variables. Skipping breakfast doesn't "cause" you to become obese. Maybe those who skip breakfast overeat at other meals or aren't as active as individuals who consistently have breakfast. Keep in mind, weight loss or weight gain comes down to the simple equation of calories in vs. calories out.

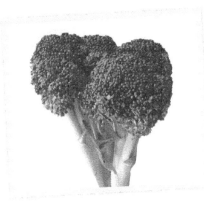

FROZEN FRUITS AND VEGGIES ARE OFTEN AS NUTRITIOUS AS FRESH ONES...

TRUE

THERE IS NO question that consuming more fruits and vegetables in our diets results in a variety of positive health benefits. It is recommended that we consume between eight and ten servings a day, but in reality most adults struggle to get half of that. Freezing fruits and vegetables for resale started to occur on a large scale basis in the mid to late 1920's, and articles written on the health aspect of these products started to appear in the early 1930's. When many people think of "fresh" fruits and vegetables, they think of what they see and buy in grocery stores. In reality, the produce sold in grocery stores may not be that fresh. Consider that produce must be picked, often before it is ripe, then sometimes stored for a day or two while chemicals are added to finish the ripening process. Finally it is transported, sometimes for thousands of miles, to a grocery store and then placed on the shelf for purchase, where again it might sit for a day or longer. This entire process

Danesi, F. and Bordoni, A. Effect of home freezing and Italian style of cooking on antioxidant activity of edible vegetables. *Journal of Food Science* (2008), Vol 73, pp. H109-H112.

can easily take one to two weeks and can lead to significant nutrient loss. In contrast, frozen fruits and vegetable are often picked at their peak of ripeness, the time when they are most nutrient packed, and frozen within hours, theoretically locking in many of those nutrients. One study which examined antioxidants in fresh and frozen vegetables was published in the *Journal of Food Science* (2008). In it the authors concluded, "the assumption that frozen vegetables have a lower antioxidant potential than fresh ones is not a universal truth, but depends on the vegetable considered" and "frozen cooked vegetables often present a higher antioxidant activity than the corresponding fresh ones." Modern flash freezing techniques can preserve the nutrition of fresh fruits and vegetables, making them available all year round.

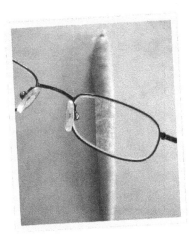

EATING CARROTS IMPROVES YOUR VISION...

FALSE

PROPOSED LINKS BETWEEN certain foods and improved eyesight have been discussed for hundreds and maybe even thousands of years. When the focus is on improving eyesight, carrots usually dominate the conversation. Many mothers and fathers have told their children to eat their carrots because it will improve their eyesight, especially in the dark. Truth be told, there is little to no evidence supporting the idea that eating carrots leads to better vision. Supposedly this myth originated during WWII when Britain's Air Ministry pilots started shooting down more Nazi bombers at night. The pilots were relying on a new technology in their war efforts, Airborne Interception Radar, but the Air Ministry didn't want the Nazis to know that. To keep their secret safe, they purposely spread a rumor that their pilots' improved vision was due to eating tremendous amounts of carrots. Carrots are high in vitamin A, which is important for good eye health; however, vitamin A

Smith, W., Mitchell, P., and Lazarus, R. Carrots, carotene and seeing in the dark. *Australian and New Zealand Journal of Ophthalmology* (1999), Vol 27, pp. 200-203.

deficiency is relatively rare in industrialized nations. Authors of one study (Smith, et al. 1999) asked people about carrot consumption and seeing in the dark. Surprisingly, they found that women in their study who said they ate more carrots reported higher rates of poor night vision. It's not likely that eating carrots negatively impacted vision in these women, but as the authors state, "it is probable that people attributing poor driving ability to their vision may be eating more carrots in the hope of reversing this decline." My wife and I have both had Lasik eye surgery so that we wouldn't need to wear contacts or glasses. If we thought we could have improved our vision by eating carrots, that would have been the first thing we would have tried!

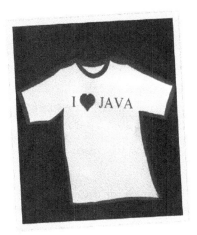

I ♥ JAVA

DRINKING COFFEE CAN HELP PREVENT TYPE II DIABETES, PARKINSON'S DISEASE, AND ALZHEIMER'S DISEASE...

TRUE

I'M VERY MUCH like 100 million or so other Americans in that I drink coffee on a regular basis. I think we all know someone who doesn't function that well in the morning until they've had two or three cups. Much to my dismay, I remember years ago hearing reports of how drinking coffee could increase the risk for cancer and heart disease. There has been a tremendous amount of research conducted on coffee. I recently performed an electronic search through the library for scientific references using the word "coffee" and came up with nearly 23,000 hits. In a nutshell, the thousands of studies conducted on coffee suggest that there are far more health benefits related to drinking coffee than there are risks. Taylor and Demmig-Adams (2007) published a review article on the health risks and benefits of coffee drinking. The authors concluded that "the most currently available evidence suggests that coffee drinking can help reduce the risk of several

---

Taylor, S. and Demmig-Adams, B. To sip or not to sip: The potential health risks and benefits of coffee drinking. *Nutrition and Food Science* (2007), Vol 37, pp. 406-418.

diseases, most notably type II diabetes, Alzheimer's disease, and Parkinson's disease although the underlying mechanisms for this effect are still being investigated." Other review articles have come up with very similar conclusions. Other studies also suggest that drinking coffee can help reduce the risk of certain cancers and even heart disease. One of the reasons coffee may be beneficial to health is that it is loaded with antioxidants. Antioxidants are molecules that help prevent healthy cells in our body from being damaged. Even with all the benefits of coffee, there can be a downside to drinking it. For some, coffee can cause the jitters or the shakes, can increase heart rate, and can result in higher levels of anxiety or nervousness. Also, those who are pregnant, have hypertension, are at risk for osteoporosis, or have epilepsy should talk to their doctors about drinking coffee.

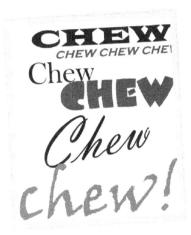

EATING MORE SLOWLY RESULTS IN CONSUMING FEWER CALORIES...

TRUE

THE TREND IN our society is to do everything in a hurry, and many Americans report that they feel rushed on a daily basis. Regretfully, this often carries over to our nutritional practices as well. I heard recently that Americans now eat one out of five meals (that's twenty percent!) in their cars. I remember, as will many of you, being scolded by my mother for eating too fast. I was the youngest of four boys. Breakfast, lunch, and dinner were by no means times to sit down, talk, and socialize as a family; they were times to eat. I imagine we looked like pigs bellying up to a trough during those meals. At times, I still find myself eating too fast and have also wondered if the speed at which we eat impacts the number of calories we consume. It looks like research is starting to address that very question. An interesting study conducted by Andrade and colleagues (2008) and published in the *Journal of the American Dietetic Association* examined number of calories

Andrade, A., Greene, G., and Melanson, K. Eating slowly led to decreases in energy intake within meals in healthy women. *Journal of the American Dietetic Association* (2008), July, pp. 1186-1191.

consumed and satiety (the feeling of being full and satisfied after a meal) in participants who either ate a meal quickly (in eight minutes) or slowly (in twenty-nine minutes). The results showed that research participants who ate fast consumed on average 645 calories whereas those who ate more slowly consumed 579 calories. Interestingly, those participants who ate more slowly also consumed more water during the meal, 409 grams of water verses 289 grams for those who ate quickly. The slower eaters also rated the meal as more satisfying and pleasant. So there appears to be a number of benefits to eating more slowly though I imagine the scolding I received from my mother for eating too fast came from a fear of my choking. One of the reasons we might eat less when we eat slowly is that it takes about twenty minutes for our bodies to signal itself when it is full. My advice is to slow down and enjoy your food; you will likely take in fewer calories.

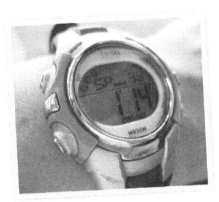

CAFFEINE IMPROVES EXERCISE PERFORMANCE...
TRUE

A MAJORITY OF people consume beverages that contain caffeine at some point during their day. For many, it's the two or three cups of coffee they drink early in the morning; for others, it comes in the form of tea, soda, or an energy drink. Individuals who purposely consume beverages that contain caffeine often say it gives them a bit of a jolt, helps them wake up or feel more awake, and gives them energy. Might this translate into improved performance when exercise or physical activity is involved? The overwhelming answer from the research that has been conducted up to this point is yes, caffeine consumption does improve exercise performance. Caffeine is considered an ergogenic aid, something that enhances performance. There has been a tremendous number of studies conducted on caffeine and performance with many of the studies showing that performance is improved by about ten percent with the aid of caffeine. Graham (2001)

Graham, T. Caffeine and exercise: Metabolism, endurance and performance. *Sports Medicine* (2001), Vol 31, pp. 785-807.

published an extensive review article on the topic in the journal *Sports Medicine* and stated that there is no doubt that caffeine enhances physical performance; he referenced many articles to support the claim. He also stated that he was not aware of any published study that has shown a negative effect of caffeine on performance. Keep in mind, though, that not everyone responds the same to caffeine. Don't assume that you can drink a cup or two of coffee and immediately knock off three or four minutes from your 5k race time or go out and bike an additional twenty miles. For some, consuming caffeine can result in getting jittery or fidgety and can contribute to increased nervousness or anxiety in others. The International Olympic Committee has set a limit on how much caffeine can be ingested by Olympic athletes. Consuming one or two cups of coffee likely wouldn't cause an athlete to be over the limit, but consuming five or six cups certainly could.

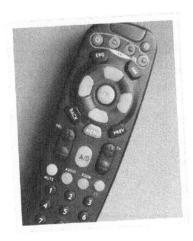

EATING WHILE WATCHING TV INCREASES CALORIC CONSUMPTION...

TRUE

WATCHING TV HAS become a routine part of our lives. Different sources report slightly different statistics on just how much TV we watch, but generally speaking, adults tend to watch two to three hours of TV a day, with children watching more like three to four hours of TV a day. Many people like to eat while watching TV, and my wife and I are no different. Like most people we live busy lives with jobs, kids, and hobbies, and watching thirty to sixty minutes of television before bed is one way we relax and unwind at night. When we watch TV, we tend to eat, and, although I am somewhat health-conscious, the food choices that I sometimes make could top the empty calorie list. Research supports the idea that we tend to eat more calories when we watch TV. Blass and colleagues (2006) did a study and reported that college students ate more pizza (thirty-six percent more calories) and more macaroni and cheese (seventy-one percent more

Blass, E., Anderson, D., Kirkorian, H., Pempek, T., Price, I., and Koleini, F. On the road to obesity: Television viewing increases intake of high-density foods. *Physiology and Behavior* (2006), Vol 88, pp. 597-604.

calories) during a thirty-minute meal while watching TV. Also, consider the types of food people generally eat while watching TV. We often choose foods like pizza, chips, cookies, and ice cream, foods that are calorie dense but nutritionally flimsy. Very rarely will you find someone sitting down and gorging themselves on broccoli, asparagus, tofu, carrots, spinach, egg whites, and tomatoes while watching TV. What can you do to try and limit the number of calories you eat in front of the TV? If you eat some or all of your meals in front of the TV, turn it off! Try to make healthier choices; eat some fruit instead of the ice cream. Finally, if you must eat things like chips, put a serving or two on a plate and put the bag back in the cupboard. That will help keep you from mindlessly eating until you hit the bottom of the bag.

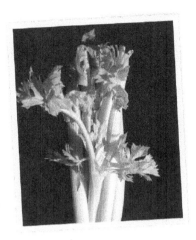

WHEN EATING CELERY, YOU BURN MORE CALORIES THAN YOU CONSUME...

FALSE

IT IS A common belief that eating certain foods results in your body burning more calories than are actually contained in the food itself. These foods are referred to as negative calorie foods. The belief revolves around the fact that when we eat food we do expend some energy breaking down and absorbing that food. This is referred to as the thermal effect of a meal (TEM), the thermal effect of eating (TEE), or diet induced thermogenesis (DIT). Celery is one of the foods that many claim to be a negative calorie food. Other foods often listed as negative calorie foods include cucumbers, mushrooms, lettuce, onions, and zucchini. When you think about it, most of these foods are basically water and fiber. With the number of people who struggle with being overweight now days, this concept of eating negative calorie foods for weight loss purposes has gotten to be popular. In fact, I did an internet search using the terms "negative calorie foods" and quickly found lots

American Dietetic Association: Food folklore: Tales and truths about what we eat. *Nutrition Now Series – Tips From the Nutrition Experts* (1999), p. 80.

of information on negative calorie diets. Apparently, when you follow this diet you can eat all the food you want, lose lots of weight, and never be hungry again. I have to admit I am very skeptical. When I read material like that, I often think back to my parents telling me the old adage "If it sounds too good to be true, it probably is." I wasn't able to find research studies that measured how many calories were burned when people ate celery or some of the other so-called negative calorie foods, but I was able to locate a book written by Registered Dietician Roberta Larson Duyff for the American Dietetic Association (1999). The author does say that the notion of eating celery as a weight loss aid because you burn more calories than it contains is a myth, and if there is a weight loss benefit it is likely because you are eating the celery in place of higher calorie foods.

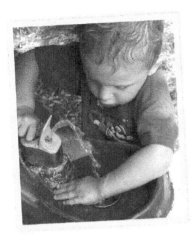

IF YOU WAIT TO DRINK UNTIL YOU ARE THIRSTY, YOU ARE ALREADY DEHYDRATED...

FALSE

I USUALLY GET thirsty two or three times during a normal day. If it is a weekend and I am at home working in the yard or the garden or playing sports with my three children, I might actually experience thirst a half dozen or more times during the day. Should I be afraid that I am chronically dehydrated and that my health is at risk? Most experts are now saying no. This notion that "if you wait to drink until you are thirsty you are already dehydrated" has been around for some time and is something that many people believe. However, there really is very little scientific evidence to support the idea. Heinz Valtin (2002) in an article published in *The American Journal of Physiology – Regulatory, Integrative and Comparative Physiology* states that this notion or fear of being dehydrated if you experience thirst is a myth. He writes that a rise in plasma osmolality (the proportion of materials like glucose and sodium in the blood) of two percent can elicit thirst and

Valtin, H. "Drink at least eight glasses of water a day." Really? Is there scientific evidence for "8 X 8"? *American Journal of Physiology—Regulatory, Integrative and Comparative Physiology* (2002), Vol 283, pp. 993-1004.

that a plasma osmolality increase of roughly five percent is when someone would be considered dehydrated. I spoke with one of my colleagues, Dr. Carl Foster, about this. Dr. Foster is a well-respected exercise physiologist and a past president of the American College of Sports Medicine. Dr. Foster stated that the idea of already being dehydrated if you got thirsty was a common belief eight to ten years ago and that most experts today think it is perfectly acceptable to let thirst be your guide in regard to drinking fluids. There certainly is nothing wrong with consuming fluids before you are thirsty, but it seems that our society has gotten to the point where the expected norm is to carry a water bottle everywhere you go and be sipping water every ten or fifteen minutes. I'm sure the companies that are making millions keeping us all well-hydrated will continue to be in support of that idea.

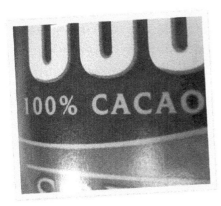

CHOCOLATE
IS GOOD FOR
YOUR HEALTH...

TRUE

ARE YOU ONE of the millions of people who love chocolate? If you are, do you sometimes feel guilty after indulging yourself? If the answer to that is yes, please keep reading! Cocoa and chocolate have been consumed for thousands of years; however, very few of us think about the health benefits associated with chocolate. In fact, it's only been recently that scientists have started paying attention to the health benefits of chocolate. Chocolate contains compounds called flavonoids, which have been shown to have antioxidant properties and be very beneficial to health. Research is starting to show that consuming chocolate may help reduce the risk of having a heart attack or stroke, aid in cancer prevention, lower blood pressure, improve insulin sensitivity, decrease blood clotting, and even improve skin health. In fact, there was a conference in 2007 in Milan, Italy, where researchers gathered to discuss current research on how chocolate consumption

Visioli, F., Bernaert, H., Corti, R., Ferri, C., Heptinstall, S., Molinari, E., Poli, A., Serafini, M., Smit, H., Vinson, J., Violi, F., and Paoletti,R. Chocolate, lifestyle, and health. *Critical Reviews in Food Science and Nutrition* (2009), Vol 49, pp. 299-312.

impacts health. Visioli, et al. (2009) published an article in the journal *Critical Reviews in Food Science and Nutrition* summarizing research presented at the conference. These authors concluded that "while the near entirety of experimental data indicate healthful consequences of cocoa intake, the caloric load of chocolate should not be overlooked and its consumption is to be positioned within a balanced and isocaloric diet." Translated, the authors are saying that chocolate is good for you, but be careful of the calories. Keep in mind that dark chocolate is much higher in flavonoid content than milk chocolate, which may contain few of these compounds as they can be destroyed during processing. Interestingly, even a quarter or a half an ounce of dark chocolate per day will likely improve health. Go ahead and indulge yourself, but remember, the darker the chocolate the better, and enjoy in moderation.

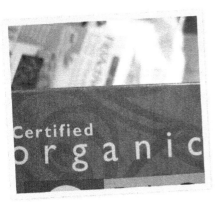

ORGANIC FOOD IS MORE NUTRITIOUS THAN NON-ORGANIC FOOD...

FALSE

A FEW HOURS before I wrote this section of the book I was in our family's garden picking raspberries with my eleven-year-old son. We ended up picking almost two pints of berries and probably ate a pint between us as we worked. Following the raspberry harvest we drifted over to the peas and simply smiled at each other as we crunched away, consuming pod and all. Growing healthy food is a topic I am very interested in, and because we rarely use chemicals in our garden, I guess I would consider myself an organic gardener. The organic food industry is one that has grown tremendously over the past five to ten years and probably will approach the fifty billion dollar mark this year. Organic farms have traditionally been small scale operations; however, as the interest in organic food increases, so does the size of the farms. Generally speaking, organic foods are grown without using things like pesticides and herbicides (for plant products) or hormones (for animal

Dangour, A., Dodhia, S., Hayter, A., Allen, E., Lock, K., and Uauy, R. Nutritional quality of organic foods: A systematic review. *American Journal of Clinical Nutrition* (2009), Vol 90, pp. 680-685.

products), and some say that organic growing processes have less of a negative impact on the environment. Many people believe that organically grown food is nutritionally superior to conventionally grown food, but research really doesn't support that. Dangour and colleagues (2009) published a review article in which they identified 162 articles on organic farming. They then determined that fifty-five were of satisfactory quality to include in their review. These authors stated that "One broad conclusion to draw from this review is that there is no evidence to support the selection of organically produced foodstuffs over conventionally produced foodstuffs to increase the intake of specific nutrients or nutritionally relevant substances." There may be many good reasons to grow or purchase organic food; however, to do so because of the belief that they contain more nutrients doesn't appear to be one of them.

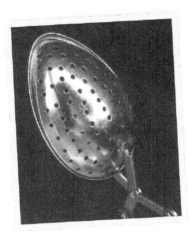

DRINKING TEA HAS MANY HEALTH BENEFITS...

TRUE

MILLIONS OF PEOPLE enjoy drinking tea, the second most consumed beverage on the planet. Until recently I had always been a heavy coffee drinker, but I had not given tea a try. Then one evening when I had a sore throat, a friend recommended that I try some throat-coat tea. I don't remember exactly what type of tea it was, but it worked and I was hooked. I still drink two or three cups of coffee in the morning, but instead of continuing to drink coffee when I get to work, I now drink tea. I really love the variety of teas on the market. I'm more of a fruity/flavored tea drinker; the two flavors I have in my office right now are "Wild Berry Zinger" and "Pomegranate Pizzazz." I spent some time on the internet investigating whether there are health benefits associated with drinking tea and found hundreds of proposed benefits. Supposedly, tea helps with hydration, memory, blood pressure, digestion, metabolism, and immunity; it curbs irritability, headaches, cardiovascular

Gupta, J., Siddique, Y., Beg, T., Ara, G., and Afzal, M. A review on the beneficial effect of tea polyphenols on human health. *International Journal of Pharmacology* (2008), Vol 4, pp. 314-338.

disease, the flu, cavities, arthritis, Parkinson's, and even bad breath! I then looked for something more scientific on the topic and found an article by Gupta and colleagues (2008) on the beneficial effects of tea published in the *International Journal of Pharmacology*. These authors cited over two hundred references in their paper and discussed how tea benefits cancer prevention, skin and cardiovascular health, and the nervous system; it can even promote weight loss. The authors stated that "research conducted in recent years reveals that both black and green teas have very similar beneficial attributes in lowering the risk of many human diseases, including several types of cancer and heart disease." There are few if any downsides to drinking tea; however, some tea does contain caffeine, so be careful if you react negatively to caffeine. If you currently don't drink tea, starting to do so would likely be a simple way to improve your health.

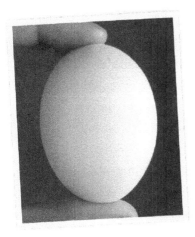

EATING PROTEIN INCREASES YOUR METABOLISM MORE THAN CARBOHYDRATES...

TRUE

COULD LOSING WEIGHT be as easy as increasing the amount of protein you eat? I do a fair amount of reading when it comes to nutrition and have to say it can be very confusing to try and figure out how much protein we should be eating. If you read bodybuilding and power lifting magazines, it is common to see recommendations that we should be taking in one or two grams of protein per pound of body weight. On the other hand, many nutritionists and registered dietitians say that we Americans take in more protein than we need. Whether we get too much or not enough protein, the question of whether protein increases our metabolism more than fats or carbohydrates is an interesting one—a question that is getting more attention these days. It turns out that protein actually does increase our metabolism more than fat or carbohydrates do. In a review article published in the *Journal of the American College of Nutrition*, Halton and Hu (2004)

Halton, T., and Hu, F. The effects of high protein diets on thermogenesis, satiety, and weight loss: A critical review. *Journal of the American College of Nutrition* (2004), Vol 23, pp. 373-385.

examined previous studies that looked at whether protein increased the thermic effect of food, which they described as being the energy required for digestion, absorption, and disposal of ingested nutrients. It is generally accepted that the thermic effect of protein is twenty to thirty percent, compared to five to ten percent for carbohydrates and zero to three percent for fat. Halton and Hu concluded that "convincing evidence exists that protein exerts an increased thermic effect when compared to fat and carbohydrate. The increased amount of energy attributable to this thermic effect is probably too small to have a visible effect on weight loss in the short term, but over periods of months or years, this difference may become significant, both clinically and statistically." So even though your body will burn more calories breaking down and absorbing protein vs. carbohydrates and fats, it is not a tremendous amount and will likely have little impact on weight in the short term.

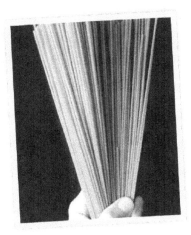

CARBOHYDRATES MAKE YOU FAT...
FALSE

OVER THE PAST ten to fifteen years there has been a sharp increase in the number of high protein, low carbohydrate diets being marketed. I believe one of the reasons so many people explore these types of diets is the mistaken belief that carbohydrates make you fat. Carbohydrates are a macronutrient; macronutrients are nutrients we need in larger quantities to help provide energy to cells for normal growth and development. Protein and fats are also macronutrients. Carbohydrates are a very important energy source for our bodies. In fact, many medical and exercise science researchers believe that carbohydrates are the preferred energy source for the brain and also are important for supplying the energy needs of muscles and other organs in the body. Various organizations recommend that you consume somewhere between forty-five and sixty-five percent of your daily calories from carbohydrates. So roughly speaking, it is recommended that

Siggaard, R., Raben, A., and Astrup, A. Weight loss during 12 weeks' ad libitum carbohydrate-rich diet in overweight and normal-weight subjects at a Danish work site. *Obesity Research* (1996), Vol 4, pp. 347-356.

the average person consume more than half of his or her daily calories in carbohydrates. If your daily caloric intake is about two thousand calories, that would mean you would want to consume roughly 250 grams of carbohydrates per day. One study published in the journal *Obesity Research* (1996) showed that subjects who ate a carbohydrate-rich, low fat diet lost more weight and fat mass than controls that did not change their diets. Additionally, it is often recommended that we consume more complex carbohydrates (whole grain pasta and vegetables) instead of simple carbohydrates (sugars). Eating too many carbohydrates certainly does have the potential to add extra pounds to your body, as does eating too many fats or proteins. Weight control really comes down to the total number of calories you consume, and a balanced diet is a healthy diet.

GENERAL HEALTH

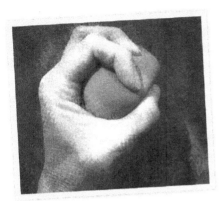

ULCERS ARE CAUSED BY STRESS...

FALSE

MANY OF US have a stereotype in our minds of the classic ulcer sufferer—overworked in a high-pressure job and over-stressed both at work and at home. Incessantly worried, they are bombarded at every side from kids, bosses, clients—the world. They eat antacids like candy and look permanently per-plexed as their troubles seem to multiply. If they could just relax and unwind, de-clutter and de-stress their lives, maybe take a stress management course, then the pain in their abdo-mens would subside, right? In the not-so-distant past, this was the advice given ulcer patients by their physicians, but as it turns out, that may not be true. Medical knowledge up until the early 1980's suggested that a decrease in blood flow to the stomach during times of anxiety weakened the stomach wall, making it vulnerable to harsh stomach acids. While stress is still thought to create an environment that is conducive to ulcers, it is no longer considered to be the primary culprit.

Freston, J. Helicobacter pylori-negative peptic ulcers: Frequency and implications for management. *Journal of Gastroenterology* (2000), Vol 35, pp. 29-32.

In the early 1980's researcher Dr. Robin Warren made a startling discovery. While conducting biopsies of ulcer patients, he found a bacterium which was later named Helicobacter pylori. Warren and his colleague, Dr. Barry Marshall, believed that this bacterium, rather than stress, was responsible for the ulcers. Because their claim was so divergent from conventional belief, it was met with much resistance and skepticism. Unable to convince his peers, Dr. Marshall set out to prove the theory in a radical way. He actually ingested some H. pylori bacteria. Days afterward, he became pale and lethargic and had, indeed, developed an ulcer. Ulcer research thereafter was focused on these bacteria. According to his article in the *Journal of Gastroenterology*, James Freston (2000) reports that "Helicobacter pylori infection is recognized throughout the world as the most common cause of both duodenal and gastric ulcers." Although stress may aggravate certain physical conditions, it does not cause ulcers.

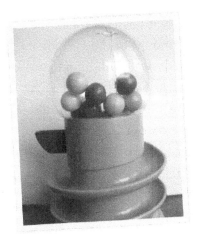

IF YOU SWALLOW GUM, IT CAN STAY IN YOUR STOMACH FOR MONTHS OR EVEN YEARS...

FALSE

MANY WERE TOLD never to do it but most did it anyway; that is they swallowed a piece of chewing gum. This may be the most perpetuated myth of all time. The parental information that is usually shared with young children to deter them from swallowing gum is that gum is not digestible (which for the most part is true) and remains in the stomach or intestines where it can turn into a huge ball of sticky goo and plug up the digestive system (which for the most part is not true). People have chewed gum type substances, usually resin from trees, for thousands and thousands of years. It wasn't until the 1840's that a businessman noticed loggers chewing tree resin and tried to mass produce and market the resin as gum but ultimately couldn't find adequate supplies of the resin. Then in the 1860's a Mexican general, with the help of a New York inventor, identified a chewing gum base that became very popular. It is this gum base which makes gum chewy and which is not

Milov, D., Andres, J., Erhart, N., and Bailey, D. Chewing gum bezoars of the gastrointestinal tract. *Pediatrics* (1998), Vol 102, pp. e22.

broken down in the system. Ultimately it passes through the digestive system in about the same amount of time as other ingested materials. It is reported that swallowing gum can result in adverse effects such as diarrhea, gas, and stomach discomfort (Milov, et al. 1998). These authors even reported the cases of three children who had masses of gum removed from their digestive system. However, in one of these reported cases a one-and-a-half-year-old girl had swallowed a number of coins that were entangled with the gum, and the two other cases were of four-year-old children who habitually swallowed five or more pieces of gum a day. So even though there are reported cases of masses of gum being removed from the intestinal tracts of children, these cases are extremely rare and usually involve large quantities of swallowed gum.

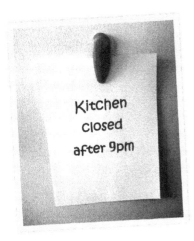

Kitchen
closed
after 9pm

YOU SHOULD NOT EAT AFTER 9:00 P.M. BECAUSE THOSE CALORIES ARE USUALLY STORED AS FAT...

FALSE

IN PAST GENERATIONS many families held to a consistent dinnertime. Now, the typical evening of the American family is much more complicated. It often involves parents chauffeuring one or more of their children to extracurricular activities and events, making it difficult to eat at the traditional dinner hour. In an article entitled "Impact of the Daily Meal Pattern on Energy Balance," France Bellisle states, "The development of the obesity epidemic has coincided with the loosening of traditional meal patterns, and it seems legitimate to ask whether this has any impact on the energy balance of individuals and their ability to control weight." Specifically, there is a question of whether eating late at night contributes to weight gain because of how the body treats those calories. There is a common misconception among many that calories eaten in the evening (say at 9:00 or 10:00 p.m.) are more readily stored as fat. It seems completely logical that food eaten

Bellisle, F. Impact of the daily meal pattern on energy balance. *Scandinavian Journal of Nutrition* (2004), Vol 48, pp. 114-118.

in the morning will be burned up by our daily activities while calories consumed just before bedtime will not have the same opportunity and, therefore, be turned into fat. There are times when even health professionals have perpetuated this popular myth. However, I could find no evidence in the medical or nutritional literature that would suggest that the body digests and stores calories any differently in the morning or at night. Most nutrition experts agree that what is important is the number of total calories eaten per twenty-four hour period, regardless of the time at which they are eaten. The question may not be when are we eating, but how much are we eating? It really gets down to calories in vs. calories out. Simply put, if you consume more calories than you burn, you will gain weight. If you burn more calories than you consume, you will lose weight. It is a simple equation but certainly a challenge to meet.

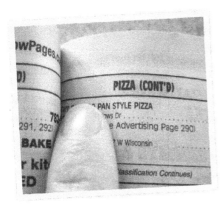

MARIJUANA GIVES YOU THE MUNCHIES...

TRUE

MARIJUANA (ALSO KNOWN as Cannabis) has been grown and consumed for thousands of years. There are reports that marijuana was used as early as 300 AD in India to help stimulate the appetite in individuals who for whatever reason had lost the desire to eat. Keep in mind that using marijuana is illegal unless prescribed by a physician (currently thirteen states have legalized medical marijuana use). Marijuana has been shown to be an analgesic (pain reducer), has been used in the treatment of glaucoma (lowers intraocular pressure), and helps relieve nausea and vomiting. Early studies that were conducted in the 1930's which examined whether marijuana stimulated appetite were not always high quality studies. However, as the recreational use of marijuana increased in the 1960's, so did the interest in conducting high quality studies (e.g., studies that used control groups and attempted to standardize the doses of marijuana consumed). Most of the

Cota, D., Marsicano, G., Lutz, B., Vicennati, V., Stalla, G., Pasquali, R., and Pagotta, U. Endogenous cannabinoid system as a modulator of food intake. *International Journal of Obesity* (2003), Vol 27, pp. 289-301.

studies conducted support the idea that marijuana does in fact give you the munchies (stimulates appetite). The authors of one study (Cota, et al. 2003), which was published in the *International Journal of Obesity*, state, "Despite the public concern related to the abuse of marijuana and its derivates, scientific studies have pointed to therapeutic potentials of Cannabinoid compounds and have highlighted their ability to stimulate appetite, especially for sweet and palatable food." This may be why marijuana use is thought to be helpful for patients with decreased appetites due to illnesses such as AIDS or late stage cancer, and it may be the reason people joke about taking late night runs to Taco John's after using marijuana. It is believed that the active ingredient in marijuana (THC) is similar to chemicals in the body which are released when your stomach is empty with the purpose of telling the brain that it is time to eat.

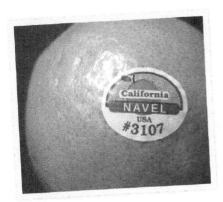

PESTICIDE RESIDUES ON FOODS CAUSE CANCER...

FALSE

THERE IS NO question that pesticides are dangerous. After all, the purpose of pesticides is to kill pests. Millions of people each year get sick from pesticide exposure, and thousands are killed. However, most of those who get sick do so because they work with the production, transportation, or application of pesticides and not because they are exposed to pesticides on the foods they eat. Some people take the idea of pesticide residue on foods very seriously. I realized this one afternoon as I watched a woman at a park rinse and carefully wipe off grapes one by one before she ate them. I think it would be fair to say that many people believe that pesticide residue on food increases their risk for cancer. Pesticides are strictly regulated. The Environmental Protection Agency sets safety standards, known as tolerances, for how much pesticide residue can be on foods. The California Department of Pesticide Regulation (CDPR) reports that most crops are treated with pesticides.

Gold, L., Stern, B., Slone, T., Brown, J., Manley, N. and Ames, B. Pesticide residues in food: Investigation of disparities in cancer risk estimates. *Cancer Letters* (1997), Vol 117, pp. 195-207.

Those pesticides not only allow farmers to grow crops in areas that might not otherwise be suitable, but they also result in higher crop yields and extended shelf life of products. The CDPR also reports that there is no pesticide residue on about sixty percent of the produce they test and that only about one percent of their test samples have pesticide residue levels that are too high. They state that years of monitoring show that most fruits and vegetables have little or no detectable residue by the time they reach market and even less by the time they are washed and served. Lois Gold and colleagues (1997) in an article titled "Pesticide Residues in Food: Investigation of Disparities in Cancer Risk Estimates" state, "Using standard methodology and measured dietary residues in the total diet study, the estimate of excess cancer risk from average lifetime exposure to synthetic pesticide residues in the diet appears to be less than one-in-a-million for each of the ten pesticides for which adequate data were available."

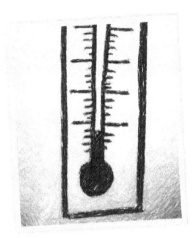

GOING OUTSIDE
WITH WET HAIR
INCREASES
YOUR CHANCE
OF CATCHING A
COLD...

FALSE

MOTHERS AND FATHERS routinely scold their children for doing things like going out in the cold without their hats and mittens on, for having their jackets unzipped, and especially for going outside with wet hair. Many parents still believe that going outside or going to sleep with wet hair increases the likelihood of catching a cold. Research going back to the 1950's has shown that this is not the case. Studies in which participants were exposed to cold viruses and then were placed in chilled or wet environments showed that the participants didn't come down with more colds than participants who were exposed to viruses in the same manner but were kept in warm or normal environments. In an article titled "Acute Cooling of the Body Surface and the Common Cold" published in the journal *Rhinology* (2002), R. Eccles writes,

There is a widely held belief that acute viral respiratory

Eccles, R. Acute cooling of the body surface and the common cold. *Rhinology* (2002), Vol 40, pp. 109-114.

infections are the result of a chill and that the onset of a respiratory infection such as the common cold is often associated with acute cooling of the body surface, especially as the result of wet clothes and hair. However, experiments involving inoculation of common cold viruses into the nose, and periods of cold exposure, have failed to demonstrate any effect of cold exposure on susceptibility to infection with common cold viruses.

Experts do agree that in order to get sick or catch a cold, you must be exposed to a virus that causes the cold. There are roughly two hundred such viruses, with rhinovirus being the culprit in the majority of cases. People often come in contact with the virus that causes a cold by breathing in viral particles after someone has sneezed or coughed or by picking up the virus from a door knob or hand rail and then touching their nose or mouth. Colds are also more common in the winter months as people tend to stay inside more and be in closer contact with one another.

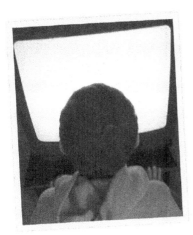

SITTING TOO CLOSE TO THE TV CAN DAMAGE YOUR VISION...

FALSE

I WOULD BE willing to wager that every single person reading this book has at one point in their childhood been instructed by their mother or father to back away from the television set, or risk going blind. It has long been thought that sitting too close to the television can damage vision. It turns out that mothers and fathers aren't the only ones who believe this falsehood. I came across one study which reported that even teachers and school children in Pakistan believed that watching television can damage vision. Many years ago some referred to the television as the radiation box. It is true that prior to 1968 televisions did emit low levels of x-rays, but I couldn't find any studies linking television watching, even back then, to eye damage. The television sets of today do not emit x-rays or any radiation. So watching *Sponge Bob* up close on Saturday morning won't damage your child's vision, but most eye experts agree that it can cause eyestrain. Signs

Toyran, M., Ozmert, E., and Yurdakok, K. Television viewing and its effect on physical health of schoolage children. *Turkish Journal of Pediatrics* (2002), Vol 44, pp. 194-203.

and symptoms of eyestrain often include red, itchy, burning, watery eyes and blurred vision. These signs and symptoms may be uncomfortable but will usually subside or disappear in an hour if one stops watching television. Think about adults who stare at a computer screen up close for far too many hours a day. I've found no evidence which would suggest that this causes eye damage either. The American Academy of Ophthalmology even reports that many kids can focus on close items better than adults. Watching television doesn't damage vision, but research (Toyran, et al. 2002) has shown that too much television viewing contributes to obesity, headaches, back pain, and sleep problems. It's probably a good idea to stay at least five feet back when watching television in order to lessen eye strain, and if you notice your child inching closer to the set, take him or her in for an eye exam as that could be an indicator of nearsightedness.

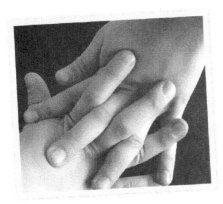

CRACKING YOUR KNUCKLES LEADS TO ARTHRITIS...

FALSE

SOME CHILDREN START cracking their knuckles because they like the cool sound it makes, some because they say it feels good, and others just because they know it annoys their parents. So what causes the "crack" or "pop" anyway? In basic terms, it's caused by air or gas bubbles being released in a joint. A more detailed explanation is offered by Castellanos and Axelrod (1990). They write, "Cracking of the knuckles results in a rapid increase of intrasynovial tension. This increased tension results in synovial fluid cavitation, which causes rapid separation of the joint and collapse of the vapour phase of the formed cavity. The consequent release of vibratory energy provides the cracking noise." No matter what causes the sound, parents have long been warning kids against knuckle cracking for fear it will lead to arthritis in old age. Only a few studies have examined whether habitual knuckle cracking leaves the "crackers" disfigured and suffering from

Castellanos, J. and Axelrod, D. Effect of habitual knuckle cracking on hand function. *Annals of the Rheumatic Diseases* (1990), Vol 49, pp. 308-309.

painful arthritis in old age. The results of these studies suggest that there is no relationship or association between cracking knuckles and arthritis. It seems reasonable to think that cracking your knuckles would lead to damage of the cartilage that covers the ends of the bones in your fingers and hands (think of the awful sound cracking your knuckles makes), but it is not true. The above-mentioned authors conducted a study in which they compared knuckle crackers vs. non-crackers and found that the crackers didn't have increased rates of arthritis in old age. They did find, however, that those who did habitually crack their knuckles were more likely to have hand swelling and decreased grip strength, and they suggest that habitual knuckle cracking should be avoided.

HAVING A SLOW METABOLISM IS A MAJOR CAUSE OF OBESITY...

FALSE

AS AN INDIVIDUAL who has worked in the area of health and wellness for many years, I've frequently heard people grumble about how thin people can eat lots of food and not gain weight and how others (usually themselves) simply need to look at something like a piece of chocolate cake and they start to gain weight and inches. Many times overweight or obese individuals blame their weight status on their "slow metabolism." However, research doesn't support the idea that being overweight or obese is the result of a slow metabolism. Dr. Donald Hensrud on MayoClinic.com states, "Yes, there is such a thing as a slow metabolism. But it's rare and it's usually not what's behind being overweight or obese—that's usually a matter of diet and exercise." In addition, Dr. Hensrud says things like genetics, family history, certain medications, lack of sleep, and unhealthy habits like skipping breakfast are more likely contributors to weight gain. Your metabolism

Goran, M. Energy metabolism and obesity. *Medical Clinics of North America* (2000), Vol 84, pp. 347-362.

(sometimes referred to as resting metabolic rate or basal metabolic rate) refers to the number of calories you burn just to keep your body working or functioning properly. Bodily functions of the heart, lungs, and digestive system as well as muscle contractions all require energy (calories). Research has also shown that overweight or obese individuals usually have a higher absolute metabolic rate as compared to thin or lean individuals simply because heavier individuals have a greater amount of body mass. When body size is taken into account, metabolic rates of obese and non-obese individuals are usually very similar. In an article entitled "Energy Metabolism and Obesity," published in *Medical Clinics of North America*, Dr. Michael Goran states that most longitudinal studies do not support the idea that reduced energy expenditure (e.g., a slow metabolism) is a significant risk factor for obesity.

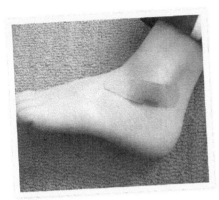

A CUT WILL HEAL FASTER IF YOU KEEP IT COVERED...

TRUE

I HAVE THE opportunity to travel a fair amount and give many talks and presentations on health myths and misconceptions. I routinely ask participants in those talks if they think it is best to uncover a wound and let it air out at certain times (e.g., when going to bed). I would say that ninety-five percent of those I ask think it is a good practice to uncover wounds and let them dry out because they think this promotes healing. It's no surprise that so many people have this misconception, as mothers and fathers have been telling their children this for years. Before researching this topic, I actually told my children the same thing. However, keeping a wound covered will keep the area moist and promote new tissue (cell) growth. Not covering a wound and having it dry out usually results in increased scab formation, which often leads to increased scarring. Scabs also slow the rate of healing because healthy regenerative tissue has a more difficult time covering a wound

Beam, J. Occlusive dressings and the healing of standardized abrasions. *Journal of Athletic Training* (2008), Vol 43, pp. 600-607.

if it is scabbed over. Keeping a wound covered also decreases the risk of infection because a covering will help keep dirt and bacteria out of the wound. Finally, a covering will help reduce the risk of re-injury. Most of us have had the unpleasant experience of having a scab tear off or have a wound re-open because it gets bumped or scraped against something. A covering can help prevent this from happening. Well-designed research studies have shown that covering a wound usually increases healing rates by three to four days. Dr. Joel Beam (2008) did a study in which he created abrasions with sandpaper on research participants (doesn't that sound like fun). Dr. Beam covered some wounds but also left some uncovered and concluded that covering wounds significantly increases healing rates. So if you've been telling your children to take bandages off their cuts and scrapes before bed, you may want to reconsider and keep those wounds covered.

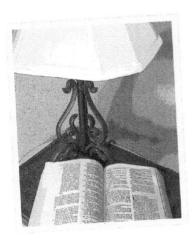

READING IN LOW LIGHT DAMAGES VISION...

FALSE

I WASN'T MUCH of a reader when I was growing up, but my children devour books like they are Willy Wonka chocolate bars. On more than one occasion I've quietly snuck up to my children's bedrooms (after the time they were supposed to be sleeping) and have discovered them reading in practical darkness next to a small nightlight or reading under their covers with flashlights. Such discoveries can worry parents. Many kids have been admonished for reading in low light conditions because their parents believe that it can damage vision. However, this has never been supported by research. In an article entitled "Myopia: The Nature Versus Nurture Debate Goes On," published in the journal *Investigative Ophthalmology and Visual Science* (1996), the authors note some environmental factors that can lead to myopia, but reading in low light conditions was not one of them. When you think about it, people used to read by candlelight by

Mutti, D., Zadnick, K., and Adams, A. Myopia: The nature versus nurture debate goes on. *Investigative Ophthalmology and Visual Science* (1996), Vol 37, 952-957.

necessity, and there is no evidence that it damaged their eyesight. Reading in low light, like sitting too close to the television, can lead to eyestrain, where the eyes can become red, irritated, watery, blurry, and dry. But eyestrain usually only lasts for a short period of time and doesn't result in vision damage. Our eyes are pretty incredible and allow us to see in a variety of environments. When in low light conditions, our eyes make a variety of adjustments to help us see better. These adjustments include pupil dilation, the production of certain chemicals to make our eyes more sensitive to light, and the nerves on the retina becoming more receptive to light. If you have to read in low light conditions, take breaks every fifteen to thirty minutes and try to remember to blink often as this will likely help reduce the chances of your eyes getting tired and irritated.

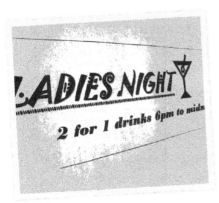

MEN HAVE
A HIGHER
TOLERANCE
FOR ALCOHOL
THAN
WOMEN...

TRUE

THIS MYTH IS very interesting. I asked a number of my friends if they thought men had a higher tolerance for alcohol, and all said no. They felt confident that men and women metabolize or oxidize alcohol the same way, at the same rate, etc. In actuality, however, men and women are different in regard to how their bodies respond to alcohol. First, men on average are a little bigger and have more body mass than women. This additional body mass may allow a greater distribution of alcohol throughout the body in men, which would then result in a slightly lower blood alcohol content. In addition to being bigger than women, men also have a greater percentage of muscle mass, which means that the water content of their bodies is higher. Men's bodies are usually fifty-five to sixty-five percent water compared to forty-five to fifty-five percent for women. Since men have a greater percentage of muscle mass, women usually have a higher percentage of body

Seitz, H., Egerer, G., Simanowski, U., Waldherr, R., Eckey, R., Agarwal, D., Goedde, H., and Von Wartburg, J. Human gastric alcohol dehydrogenase activity: Effect of age, sex, and alcoholism. *Gut* (1993), Vol 34, pp. 1433-1437.

fat compared to men. Alcohol doesn't dissolve in body fat, but it does in water. This also allows for a greater distribution of alcohol throughout a man's body and would result in slightly lowered alcohol content in the blood. Possibly the most significant difference in how men and women metabolize alcohol has to do with an enzyme called alcohol dehydrogenase (ADH). This enzyme actually starts to metabolize or break down alcohol in the stomach. More alcohol leaving the stomach will ultimately result in a higher blood alcohol content. Seitz, et al. (1993) conducted a study looking at ADH activity in men and women and concluded that "women exhibit a significant lower gastric alcohol dehydrogenase activity than men when alcohol dehydrogenase is measured at high ethanol (alcohol) concentrations." This is just another example of the many ways in which men's and women's bodies differ.

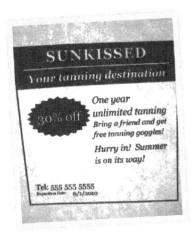

EXCESSIVE TANNING CAN DAMAGE INTERNAL ORGANS...

FALSE

IT IS NOT true that tanning, even excessive tanning, can damage internal organs. Many people falsely believe this because of a story, widely circulated on the internet, which describes a young woman trying to get a tan for her wedding. Supposedly this woman visited a number of tanning salons, with some versions of the story saying up to a dozen, a week or two before her wedding. The excessive tanning then resulted in her internal organs getting "fried," resulting in her death. As hard as I looked into the medical literature, I couldn't find a reference to this poor woman, so I feel confident saying that the incident never happened. Also consider that the rays from tanning beds don't penetrate the skin more than one six-teenth of an inch. Tanning beds expose users to light bulbs that emit ultraviolet radiation, an artificial light similar to the light you are exposed to when you are out in the sun. Indoor tanning started to become very popular in the 1970's and is

Levine, J., Sorace, M., Spencer, J., and Siegel, D. The indoor UV tanning industry: A review of skin cancer risk, health benefit claims, and regulation. *Journal of the American Academy of Dermatology* (2005), Vol 53, pp. 1038-1044

a multi-billion dollar industry today. Because of the billions spent on indoor tanning, the industry is able to hire powerful lobbyists who work hard to block indoor tanning regulations both at the state and federal levels. Currently, only about half the states in this country have regulatory laws. The tanning industry claims that tanning is safe and even beneficial to health. On the other hand, scientific and medical literature paints a much different picture. Levine and colleagues (2005) state that in recent years research has suggested an association between sun bed use (indoor tanning) and a significantly elevated risk of skin cancer. This association or correlation is supported by other researchers as well. Additional risks of indoor tanning include skin burn, allergic reaction, eye damage, wrinkles, and damage to blood vessels.

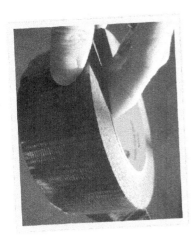

COVERING A WART WITH DUCT TAPE WILL USUALLY MAKE IT GO AWAY...

TRUE

WARTS ARE VERY common. Just this morning I had the chance to look at a common wart on the thumb of my six-year-old and a plantar wart on my wife's foot. When I was younger, my mother used to take me to the dermatologist every twelve to fifteen months to have a cluster of warts frozen or burned (with liquid nitrogen) off of my elbow. For the most part warts don't significantly impact our daily activities. My six-year-old functions just fine, and at times I think he enjoys having something readily available to pick at to help pass the time at school. My wife's plantar wart is a source of some pain and irritation; however, she was able to run a half marathon recently. Even though my warts were a source of some embarrassment during my pre-teen years, I managed to make it through without lasting psychological damage. Many people choose to have their warts removed, but about seventy percent of warts will go away on their own in one to two years

Focht, D., Spicer, C., and Fairhok, M. The efficacy of duct tape vs cryotherapy in the treatment of Verruca Vulgaris (the common wart). *Archives of Pediatric and Adolescent Medicine* (2002), Vol 156, pp. 971-974.

even without any type of treatment. Some people choose to visit their doctors to have their warts frozen or burned off, and many others purchase a variety of over-the-counter wart removers. One home remedy that appears to be successful is applying duct tape to warts. Dr. Dean Focht and colleagues (2002) did a study in which they compared using duct tape vs. freezing with liquid nitrogen. They found that at the end of the study eighty-five percent of the research participants who used duct tape had complete resolution of their warts vs. sixty percent of the participants who had their warts frozen off. The process usually involves applying duct tape over a wart for five to six days, then soaking the wart and abrading the dead skin off the wart with a pumice stone or something similar. This is to be repeated until the wart is gone. No one is sure why duct tape helps remove warts, but the current thinking is that the tape causes irritation around the wart which then stimulates the body to attack it.

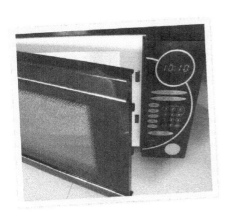

WATER HEATED IN A MICROWAVE CAN ERUPT AND CAUSE SEVERE BURNS...

MYTH 59

TRUE

THIS ONE SOUNDS a bit hard to believe, but it is true that water heated in a microwave can erupt and cause serious injury. Considering the millions of people who heat water for things like coffee and tea in microwaves, the phenomena of erupting or exploding water is rare. Think of the last time you boiled water on top of your conventional stove. Do you remember seeing small air bubbles form on the bottom and sides of the pot? Eventually these bubbles release from the surface of the pot, rise, and break the surface of the water. This is what we usually think of as "boiling"; the boiling point of water is 100 C°. When you heat water in a microwave, this normal boiling process does not occur. Rarely will you see bubbles form or boiling take place even though the water can be extremely hot. Heating water in a microwave occurs much faster than on a normal stove, and this is one of the reasons that the bubbles don't form. The absence of bubbles

Hosack, H., Marler, N., and MacIsaac, D. Microwave mischief and madness. *The Physics Teacher* (2002), Vol 40, pp. 264-266.

123

actually allows the water to heat up to more than 100° C, sometimes referred to as superheated water. In an article entitled "Microwave Mischief and Madness," Heather Hosack and colleagues (2002) write, "Superheated water will flash boil or geyser out of the container if boiling is suddenly triggered by vibration, or by an object (like a spoon) or a powder or your upper lip." Imagine if this happened while you were bringing the cup out of the microwave; it could cause the extremely hot water to erupt in your face or spill onto a nearby child. To prevent this from happening, add something to the water (e.g., sugar, wooden stir stick) before heating, let heated water sit for one to two minutes before moving, or use a container which is slightly scratched as the scratches aid in the production of bubbles.

CROSSING YOUR LEGS LEADS TO VARICOSE VEINS...

FALSE

MYTH 60

MOST PEOPLE WHO cross their legs probably do so because they feel it is a comfortable way to sit. However, people likely cross their legs for a variety of reasons in a variety of social situations. For example, some people may cross their legs when they are nervous or anxious and others because it makes them feel distinguished or sophisticated; for others crossing their legs may be a way to create a barrier and protect personal space when interacting with someone new. I often cross my legs when I am sitting in long meetings due to pure boredom. It gives me a reason to move around a little bit and helps me stay awake. Sometimes I pretend the foot I have elevated in the air is a fishing rod and I am casting for rainbow trout in a secluded mountain river in Colorado. Some people believe that crossing your legs can increase the pressure in your lower legs or block blood flow and cause varicose veins. There is no evidence that crossing your legs causes varicose

Lee, A., Evans, C., Allan, P., Ruckley, C., and Fowkes, F. Lifestyle factors and the risk of varicose veins: Edinburgh vein study. *Journal of Clinical Epidemiology* (2003), Vol 56, pp. 171-179.

veins or makes existing varicose veins worse. A varicose vein is a vein near the surface of the body that, for a variety of reasons, might begin to lose its elasticity; the walls (or sides) may begin to weaken, and blood may pool in these veins causing them to enlarge or balloon up. Roughly twenty to twenty-five percent of adults will develop varicose veins. Even though crossing the legs doesn't cause varicose veins, some people report discomfort in the ankles, knees, hips, and even low back after they sit with their legs crossed. Lee and colleagues (2003) showed that height, family history, and obesity are likely reasons people develop varicose veins. Other reasons might be pregnancy, standing for long periods, and physical inactivity. If you enjoy sitting with your legs crossed, you can do so without fear that you are causing varicose veins. Happy fishing!

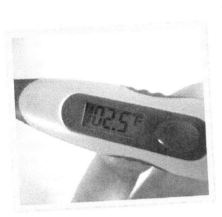

YOU SHOULD STARVE A FEVER AND FEED A COLD...

FALSE

MANY PEOPLE, INCLUDING me, get sick one or two times a year. When I'm sick I often try to remember how to appropriately treat whatever is ailing me (cold, fever, etc.) by following the common saying "starve a fever and feed a cold." However, when I'm in the middle of fighting an illness, I usually can't remember which one I should be starving and which one I should be feeding. What if you accidently "feed" or "starve" the wrong condition—will that make it worse? This idea of starving a fever and feeding a cold may be a result of the belief that colds were due to decreases in body temperature, so eating more would add calories to the body and increase temperature. On the other hand, withholding calories when you had a fever would help decrease body temperature. Also, many times when people have fevers they don't have much of an appetite; some believe that this is our body's way of telling us not to consume calories. Many people still recommend

Bazar, K., Yun, A., and Lee, P. "Starve a fever and feed a cold": Feeding and anorexia may be adaptive behavioral modulators of autonomic and T helper balance. *Medical Hypotheses* (2005), Vol 64, pp. 1080-1084.

starving fevers and feeding colds (just spend a few minutes scanning the internet to see how popular this myth is), but most reputable healthcare professions do not. The advice often heard from doctors and nurses to people who are sick include staying hydrated, resting, and eating some healthy food if you have an appetite. There is research (Bazar, et al. 2005) that suggests eating may positively impact some immune system functions in the body. But again, most healthcare professionals wouldn't recommend people forcing themselves to eat if they are feeling nauseated or if they have no appetite. The bottom line is, if you are sick you should rest, drinks fluids, and eat some healthy foods as tolerated.

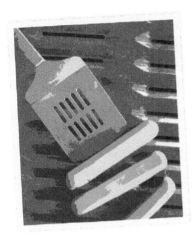

IT IS HEALTHIER TO GRILL WITH PROPANE THAN CHARCOAL...

TRUE

THERE ARE MILLIONS upon millions of people who fire up their grills every day in this country. I'm usually not one to exaggerate things, but I honestly believe that I could be given the title "World's Worst Griller." I don't even want to think about how many steaks, hamburgers, pork chops, and chicken breasts I have scorched on the grill and had to throw away. It really is like the movie Ground Hog Day because it happens over and over and over again. Usually the scenario goes something like this: I put some steaks on the grill, set the grill to medium or medium high heat, walk away to do something else for just a few minutes (e.g., pick up the yard, pick some herbs in the garden, play with the dog) and return to steaks that are on fire. One day I returned to a grill that was entirely engulfed in flames. I couldn't turn the gas off with the plastic handles on the front of the grill because they were completely melted; I had to use a fire extinguisher. Some people love grilling with

Farhadian, A., Jinap, S., Abas, F., and Sakar, Z. Determination of polycyclic aromatic hydrocarbons in grilled meat. *Food Control* (2010), Vol 21, pp. 606-610.

charcoal and others love propane, but is using one healthier than the other? It appears that the answer is yes, and it's propane. Authors of one study (Farhadian, et al. 2010) examined polycyclic aromatic hydrocarbons (PAH's), which are carcinogenic compounds. They reported that grilling with charcoal produced significantly more PAH's than grilling with propane. One reason grilling with charcoal may produce more PAH's is that charcoal usually burns hotter, so there is an increased risk of charring the meat. Some additional tips to reduce PAH's in grilled food include turning meat frequently, partially cooking meat in the microwave before grilling it, removing any burnt parts, and marinating the meat in lemon juice before cooking.

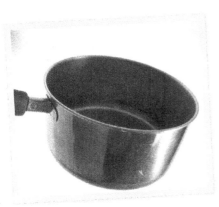

COOKING IN ALUMINUM POTS CONTRIBUTES TO ALZHEIMER'S DISEASE...

FALSE

OF ALL THE myths I've written about, the topic of whether aluminum causes Alzheimer's could be the one about which I've seen the most research. For example, when I performed a search in Google Scholar using the keywords "Alzheimer's" and "Aluminum," 21,800 articles on the topic were identified. Much of what I read doesn't support the idea that there is a direct causal link between aluminum and Alzheimer's disease. That is, being exposed to aluminum won't cause you to get Alzheimer's. However, research has shown that there are increased levels of aluminum in the brain cells of Alzheimer's patients. Again, it likely isn't the aluminum that is causing Alzheimer's; it might be that for some reason brain cells in people with Alzheimer's tend to accumulate more aluminum. In an article in the *Journal of Alzheimer's Disease*, Perl and Moalem (2006) write, "It is highly unlikely that aluminum represents an etiologic agent for Alzheimer's disease." However

Perl, D. and S. Moalem. Aluminum and Alzheimer's disease, a personal perspective after 25 years. *Journal of Alzheimer's Disease* (2006), Vol 9, pp. 291-300.

they do say that aluminum could play a role in the process leading to the disease. Aluminum is the third most abundant element on earth; we are exposed to trace amounts of aluminum every day when we breathe, eat, and drink. Most of the aluminum that enters our bodies is excreted. If small amounts of aluminum were toxic to humans, we would all be in big trouble! The focus of this particular myth is whether cooking in aluminum pots contributes to Alzheimer's. Because the aluminum exposure caused by cooking in aluminum pots is very, very small and because most of the aluminum that enters our bodies is excreted, the logical conclusion is that it does not. My wife and I are crazy about popcorn; we eat it almost every night. A few years ago we bought an aluminum popcorn maker. If I thought there was even a remote chance that using this popcorn maker could contribute to Alzheimer's, it would have been thrown out a long time ago.

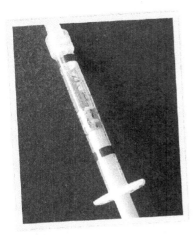

THE FLU SHOT CAN CAUSE THE FLU...

FALSE

EVERY YEAR THE flu season comes around, and every year you have to make a decision of whether or not you are going to get vaccinated. If you have children, you also need to decide if you will get them vaccinated. Trust me when I say that can be a traumatic experience! I've also learned that flu shots can be a very sensitive issue for lots of people. The Centers for Disease Control and Prevention (CDC) estimate that roughly 200,000 people are hospitalized and 36,000 people die from the flu annually. The CDC offers a great deal of information about the flu as well as information about the types of flu vaccines offered. There basically are two types of flu vaccines available. The first is the flu shot, sometimes referred to as trivalent inactivated influenza vaccine. The flu shot is considered "inactivated" because it contains killed flu viruses. The second type of vaccine is the flu mist or nasal spray. You will sometimes see this type of vaccine referred

Tosh, P., Boyce, T., and Poland, G. Flu myths: Dispelling the myths associated with live attenuated influenza vaccine. *Mayo Clinic Proceedings* (2008), Vol 1, pp. 77-84.

to as live attenuated influenza vaccine. The spray or mist is considered "live" because it contains live, but weakened, flu viruses. Both vaccines have been approved by the Food and Drug Administration, and neither of the vaccines will result in your getting the flu. The live attenuated vaccine is newer (only commercially available since about 2003) than the inactivated vaccine; however, some people can be hesitant to get the flu spray or mist because they are worried about the "live but weakened" nature of the vaccine. A very well-written article by Tosh, et al. (2008) describes how the live attenuated vaccine is both a safe and effective vaccine. So why do you sometimes feel like you get the flu after you get a flu shot? The body can sometimes experience an immune response to a flu shot which can result in flu-like symptoms. These symptoms can include muscle aches, headache, fever, cough, and a sore throat, but they are generally mild and only last two or three days—much less serious than the actual flu.

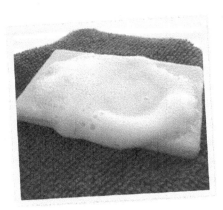

ANTIBACTERIAL SOAP IS SUPERIOR TO REGULAR SOAP IN PREVENTING ILLNESSES...

FALSE

ANTIBACTERIAL SOAPS HAVE become incredibly popular over the past five to ten years. It can be a bit overwhelming to walk down the soap aisle at your shopping market and see all of the antibacterial soap choices available. Roughly between seventy and seventy-five percent of soaps available for purchase have "antibacterial" someplace on the label. This, as well as wording like "kills up to 99.9% of bacteria," may help explain why these soaps have grown in popularity. But the question still remains—are antibacterial soaps any better at killing germs than good old-fashioned soap and water? Most of the research on the topic is suggesting "no." Allison Aiello and colleagues (2007) published a review article in the journal *Clinical Infectious Diseases* in which they examined the results of twenty-seven studies on this topic. The authors concluded, "Collectively, the microbiological efficacy studies strongly suggest that concentrations of triclosan used in consumer

Aiello, A., Larson, E., and Levy, S. Consumer antibacterial soaps: Effective or just risky? *Clinical Infectious Diseases* (2007), Vol 45, pp. S137-S147.

liquid hand soaps do not provide a benefit over plain soap for reducing bacterial levels found on the hands." Triclosan is the major antibacterial agent in antibacterial soaps. There are even some studies that suggest triclosan may contribute to resistant strains of bacteria and kill healthy bacteria on the skin. Additionally, in 2005 an FDA advisory group studied this topic and came to the conclusion that there is no evidence that antibacterial soap is superior to regular soap. It certainly is important to wash our hands, especially when we are sick, if we are cooking and handle raw meat, and after we go to the bathroom. However, most of us do a pretty horrible job when it comes to washing our hands. Proper hand washing technique calls for first wetting the hands, lathering the hands with soap for a minimum of twenty seconds, and then rinsing for another ten seconds. Next time you wash your hands, see how long it really takes you!

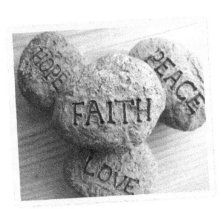

CONSISTENTLY ATTENDING RELIGIOUS SERVICES INCREASES LIFE EXPECTANCY...

TRUE

ON MOST SUNDAY mornings our household is as busy as a beehive. Getting kids up and fed, teeth and hair brushed, clothes on without stains or holes—it's no small task! I'm sure many of you with children can relate. Our family goes through this routine to get ready for church almost every Sunday morning, not because we think it will prolong our lives, but because it is something we want to do, and we enjoy it. However, a large body of research is now suggesting that attending religious services positively impacts longevity (how long we live). McCullough and colleagues (2000) published a study in the journal *Health Psychology* in which they examined data from forty-two samples or studies that looked at religious involvement and death rates. By comparing their data at various follow-up points of the study, they found that people who rated themselves as being highly religious were about thirty percent more likely to be alive than those who were less religious. The

McCullough, M., Larson, D., Hoyt, W., and Koenig, H. Religious involvement and mortality: A meta-analytic review. *Health Psychology* (2000), Vol 19, pp. 211-222.

authors concluded that "although the correlational nature of the data prohibit causal inferences, religious involvement has a nontrivial, favorable association with all-cause mortality." In other words, attending religious services doesn't necessarily cause you to live longer, but there appears to be a relationship or association between the two variables. It is well known that people with stronger social ties live longer and are generally healthier people. This certainly could contribute to why people who attend religious services live longer. Other contributing factors might be that people who attend religious services tend to engage in less risky behaviors such as smoking, drinking, and doing drugs; they may tend to watch out for each other, have less stress, and be better able to cope with traumatic events in their lives. Another possible reason might be that established routines and rituals in people's lives give them something to look forward to as well as a sense of meaning and purpose.

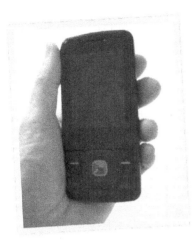

CELL PHONE USAGE HAS BEEN LINKED TO BRAIN TUMORS...

TRUE

THE QUESTION OF whether cell phone usage increases the risk of brain tumors is one that I have been following for a few years. The majority of studies that I have read or websites that I have visited (e.g., Center for Disease Control) have usually concluded that there doesn't appear to be a link between the two. However, up to this point there has been a lack of long-term data, that is research on people who have been using cell phones for ten plus years. Khurana and colleagues (2009) published a recent review article in which they examined eleven long-term studies on the topic. They concluded that "the long-term epidemiologic data suggest an increased risk of being diagnosed with an ipsilateral brain tumor related to cell phone usage of ten years or more." Ipsilateral means that the tumor is on the same side of the head as where the phone is usually held. So it appears that research is starting to point to a connection between long-term use of cell phones

Khurana, V., Teo, C., Kundi, M., Hardell, L., and Carlberg, M. Cell phones and brain tumors: A review including the long-term epidemiologic data. *Surgical Neurology* (2009), Vol 72, pp. 205-215.

and brain tumors. Cell phones use small amounts of radiation to send signals to cell towers which allows users to complete calls. How much radiation one is exposed to (keep in mind that we are talking about small amounts) can depend on the brand of phone, time spent using the phone, and distance from the nearest cell tower. Cell phones became popular in the 1990's and continue to gain in popularity. Khurana and colleagues (2009) also state that there are three billion cell phone users around the world. The message that there is a possible link between cell phones and brain tumors may be starting to spread. Currently a number of states in the U.S. are considering legislation that would require warning labels on cell phones, and it is getting more common to read recommendations like using a wired earpiece with cell phones or texting instead of making calls, so that the phone is not next to your head. But please don't text while driving!

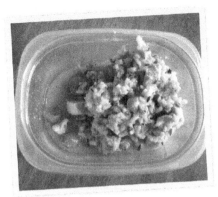

THERE IS A LINK BETWEEN EATING OUT OF PLASTIC CONTAINERS THAT CONTAIN BPA AND GETTING CANCER...

TRUE

I DON'T BELIEVE in spending tremendous amounts of money on fancy Tupperware containers. If you were to look inside my refrigerator, you would likely see leftovers placed in old plastic margarine, cottage cheese, Cool Whip, and yogurt containers. Many times when I'm in a hurry and want a quick snack, I'll take out one of these containers with leftovers in it and be tempted to toss it into the microwave for thirty or forty-five seconds. I actually did that a couple of years ago, and in less than a minute the container I was using turned into a twisted, melted mess. Much of the health concern revolving around microwaving in plastic containers is related to bisphenol A (BPA), a chemical used when plastics are made. BPA is known as an endocrine disruptor, which means that it interferes with the creation and use of hormones in the body. Most of us have enough problems; we don't need another thing messing with our hormones. Over the past few years there has

Vogel, S. The politics of plastics: The making and unmaking of bisphenol A "safety." *American Journal of Public Health* (2009), Vol 99, pp. S559-S566.

been greater concern about eating and drinking out of containers that contain BPA. Some products are now starting to share information like "BPA free" on their label, and recently Canada classified BPA as toxic. Studies have shown that various components of plastic containers can leach out into food when they are heated. Many of these studies have shown that the amount is small and usually falls within acceptable standards; however, more current research is starting to paint a slightly different picture. In a recent article published in the *American Journal of Public Health* (2009), Sarah Vogel states, "New research on very-low-dose exposure to BPA suggests an association with adverse health effects, including breast and prostate cancer, obesity, neurobehavioral problems, and reproductive abnormalities. These findings challenge the long-standing scientific and legal presumption of BPA's safety."

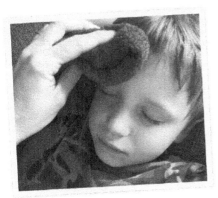

YOU SHOULD
USUALLY LET
FEVERS RUN
THEIR COURSE
WITHOUT
GIVING
MEDICATIONS...

TRUE

A FEVER OCCURS when our core body temperature is higher than it is supposed to be. Normally, our body temperature hovers around 98.6 degrees F, but it is common for that number to fluctuate a degree or so during the day. Usually, our temperature is at its lowest point sometime in the early morning and at its highest point sometime in the late afternoon. Our temperature will also rise during periods of increased physical activity. Many consider the temperature of 100.5 degrees F to be the point where we officially have a fever. My wife and I are parents of three children, and I can tell you that the first time one of our kids had a fever, we panicked. What is wrong? What if the fever keeps going up? When should we go to the doctor? What can we do to lower the fever? How long before brain cells start dying? What we experienced is common and is sometimes referred to as fever phobia. Generally speaking, fever phobia is the fear that something bad is happening

Glatstein, M. and Scolnik, D. Fever: To treat or not to treat. *World Journal of Pediatrics* (2008), Vol 4, pp. 245-247.

when someone (e.g., your child) has a fever. As parents, our first desire with a sick child is to treat and take care of him or her. When a fever is involved, many think that this means doing something to lower it. However, experts say that is not what we should usually do. It turns out that a fever is part of our body's natural immune system defense against invading microorganisms. Glatstein and Scolnik (2008) published an article entitled "Fever: To Treat or Not to Treat" in the *World Journal of Pediatrics*. The authors state, "In humans, increased temperature is associated with decreased microbial reproduction and increased inflammatory response." Both help us fight invading viruses and bacteria. The authors also state that "since fever is not in itself harmful, and might even be protective, there is no particular reason to treat it other than as a comfort measure."

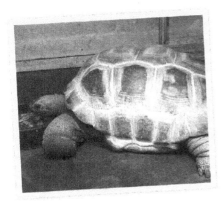

TOUCHING REPTILES AND AMPHIBIANS INCREASES YOUR RISK OF CONTRACTING A SALMONELLA INFECTION...

TRUE

ONE OF OUR family's favorite summertime activities is to get in our canoe and float down a river that is not too far from our house. The float usually covers four to six miles, and we make frequent stops along sandbars to play football, swim, roast hotdogs, build sand castles, and, of course, search for animals. Our three boys always view these trips as mini-adventures, and they are continually on the lookout for critters. They commonly find snakes, frogs, turtles, and toads and are never bashful about playing with them. It hasn't been until recently that I've learned that handling reptiles and amphibians can increase your risk of contracting a salmonella infection. People often associate salmonella infections with eating contaminated foods like chicken or eggs. However, it is true that you can get a salmonella infection from reptiles and amphibians. The Centers for Disease Control and Prevention

Mermin, J., Hutwagner, L., Vugia, D., Shallow, S., Daily, P., Bender, J., Koehler, J., Marcus, R., and Angulo, F. Reptiles, amphibians, and human salmonella infection: A population-based, case-control study. *Clinical Infectious Diseases* (2004), Vol 38, pp. S253-261.

also says that birds, cats, horses, and even dogs can pass salmonella in their feces. Mermin and colleagues (2004) performed a study to estimate the burden of reptile- and amphibian-associated salmonella infections and published it in the journal *Clinical Infectious Diseases*. The authors concluded that reptile and amphibian exposure is associated with about 74,000 salmonella infections every year in the United States. The authors also stated that their findings "emphasize the need for improved prevention efforts without which thousands of preventable cases of reptile- and amphibian-associated salmonellosis may continue to occur annually in the United States." If you are interested in decreasing your or your family's risk of contracting a salmonella infection, avoid contact with reptiles and amphibians (especially for young children) or thoroughly wash hands after doing so.

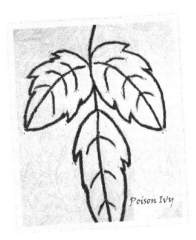

Poison Ivy

YOU CAN CATCH POISON IVY FROM SOMEONE ELSE'S RASH...

FALSE

SOME PEOPLE AVOID spending time outdoors in the summer for fear of coming in contact with poison ivy. I consider myself to be pretty lucky in that I've never had severe reactions to poison ivy. I do spend many hours outdoors hiking, cutting wood, mountain biking, and walking to secret fishing holes. I don't remember ever getting poison ivy as a child, but every so often as an adult I'll get a slight rash after exposure. Even though my reactions tend to be what I would categorize as minor, the small spots that appear can be intensely itchy and can blister up after a few days. Poison ivy reactions occur after coming in contact with urushiol oil on the leaves, stem, or roots of the poison ivy plant. Since the oil is found in the stem and roots, it is possible to get a rash from poison ivy even during colder months of the year. It is also recommended not to burn poison ivy plants as breathing or coming in contact with the smoke can lead to a reaction. The rash that occurs

Jackson Allen, P. Leaves of three, let them be: If it were only that easy! *Dermatology Nursing* (2006), Vol 18, pp. 236-242.

after exposure can get very red and irritated and can blister up. The blisters often break and leak fluid. This is not a pretty sight, and I can see how some might think they could spread or catch poison ivy from these rashes. However, that is not the case. In an article written in *Dermatology Nursing*, Patricia Jackson Allen writes, "The rash may grow in size and development of new vesicles can occur during the first 2 weeks without additional contact with urushiol due to the allergenic response of the host. This leads to the common belief that the serum from vesicles is allergenic. The serum released from the vesicles is not antigenic and does not spread the allergic contact reaction." It is probably good practice to avoid other people's poison ivy rashes and the fluid oozing out of them. But in the unlikely event that contact should occur, you can feel confident that you won't soon be developing a rash of your own.

NON-HEALTH MYTHS

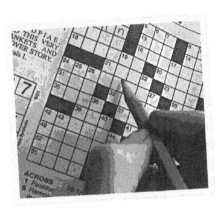

AMERICANS HAVE MORE FREE TIME TODAY THAN THEY DID IN 1965...

TRUE

WE'VE ALL HAD our share of those days when we've felt like we couldn't get everything accomplished that needed to be done, much less have any free time. However, research suggests that we actually have gained about five hours of free time per week since the 1960's (Robinson and Godbey 1997). It is interesting that even though the amount of free time we have has increased, most Americans state that they feel more rushed and they think they actually have less free time. So what is considered free time? Most researchers would consider things like watching TV, listening to music, reading, socializing, and engaging in hobbies, recreational activities, sports, adult education, and even religious activities as free time. Essentially, things you do in your free time are completely your own choice. Think of free time activities as those that are not essential to your life or survival. Things you might do that would not be considered free time would include sleeping,

Robinson, J. and Godbey, G. *Time for Life: The Surprising Ways Americans Use Their Time.* Pennsylvania State UP: University Park, PA, 1997.

eating, grooming, taking care of your kids, doing housework, and working at a job that pays you wages. Contrary to what some might believe, checking your friend's status on Facebook and watching TV are not essential to survival. Robinson and Godbey also state that 1) middle aged, college-educated, married parents, where both spouses work have the least amount of free time, 2) people in urban areas have about one hour more per week of free time compared to those in rural areas, and 3) we have nearly forty hours of free time per week (five hours each weekday, six hours on Saturday, and over seven hours on Sunday). Most people overestimate how much time they spend at work and underestimate how much free time they have. It's not uncommon for someone to say that they are very busy and that they don't have time for things like exercise, yet they will watch three or four hours of TV a day!

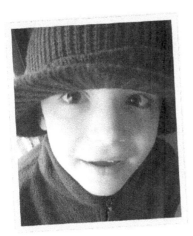

WEARING A TIGHT HAT LEADS TO HAIR LOSS...

FALSE

HAIR LOSS CAN be a traumatic experience for men and women. Right or wrong, our society places a great deal of emphasis on appearance, and many people take pride in having a thick, full head of hair. Hair loss is common in later life, especially among men; however, many individuals start to experience hair loss in their early to mid twenties. The hair care industry is a multi-billion dollar industry, and a significant portion of the money spent on hair care is spent on products related to hair loss. Discussions on hair loss have been occurring for a long time. I ran across an interesting article entitled "The Prophylaxis of Baldness," published in the *Journal of the American Medical Association* in 1903. Our understanding of the cause of hair loss is different today than it was in the early 1900's. It is not true that wearing a hat, even a tight hat, contributes to hair loss. Some have speculated that this myth came about after men who entered the military noticed that they started to lose their hair shortly after enlisting. Many of these men felt their hair loss was related to wearing tight military hats and helmets. In reality, their hair loss likely would have started to occur whether they joined the military or not. I read a large number of articles that addressed the causes of hair loss. These articles identified factors such as genetics, skin diseases, nutrition, trauma, medications, and endocrine disorders as legitimate contributors to hair loss. However, not a single article mentioned the dangers of wearing hats. An article published in *Consumer Reports on Health* (2007) stated, "This myth may have arisen in part because people often wear hats to cover their balding heads. And tight hats do not restrict blood flow in the scalp sufficiently to harm the hair follicles." If you for some reason enjoy wearing tight hats, you can enjoy doing so without fear of losing your hair.

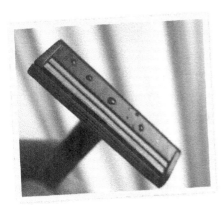

SHAVING MAKES HAIR GROW BACK THICKER...

FALSE

MYTH 74

MANY YEARS AGO when I was in middle school, one of my best friends helped himself to one of his father's razors and a can of shaving cream and started shaving his chest. He told me that he had heard from someone in high school (always a reliable source of valid health information) that shaving causes hair to grow. After a few weeks of shaving one to two times a day and seeing no results, he abandoned his quest to speed up the process of entering into manhood. There are a number of interesting reasons why people might believe that shaving causes hair to grow back thicker. First, the base of hair or the part closest to the skin is the thickest. So following shaving, some might mistakenly think that their hair actually appears thicker. Additionally, after you shave, the stubble has a blunt end or tip which can be rough (hence the term stubble) and give the appearance of being thicker. Some have even speculated that another factor that may have contributed to

Lynfield, Y. and MacWilliams, P. Shaving and hair growth. *The Journal of Investigative Dermatology* (1970), Vol 55, pp. 170-172.

this myth is the fact that when we first start to shave when we are young, our hair is relatively thin, but it gets slightly thicker (this occurs naturally) as we get older. However this is not due to shaving. Finally, hair might actually appear slightly darker following shaving as the dark stubble is contrasted against the skin. Research on shaving and hair growth dates back to the 1920's and does not support the idea that shaving causes hair to grow back thicker. Lynfield and MacWilliams (1970) conducted a study in which they examined whether shaving impacted the weight, length, and width of hair. These authors concluded that "No significant differences in rate of hair growth, either in length or weight, and no coarsening of individual hairs could be ascribed to shaving." This is obviously bad news to middle school students everywhere!

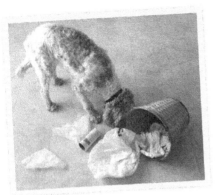

A DOG'S MOUTH IS CLEANER THAN A HUMAN'S...

FALSE

MY WIFE AND I have always had dogs, and at times we have had up to three of them. So we have plenty of stories of the interesting things dogs eat and do with their mouths. For example, one day I had our cute little Cavachon (Scout) on a walk out in the woods on a sunny winter day. The snow was fairly deep, so we followed deer trails as we walked. I'd estimate that by the time we completed our two hour walk, Scout had consumed his body weight in deer droppings. He devoured those little delicacies like I devour chocolate covered coffee beans. On another occasion in the summer, he emerged from under a bush with a bird carcass that was badly decomposed and rancid. Given their eating habits, is it even remotely possible that a dog's mouth could be cleaner than a human's? The simple answer is no. This myth may have come about because people frequently see dogs lick their wounds, wounds which rarely get infected. It's possible that

Rayan, G., Downard, D., Cahill, S., and Flourney, D. A comparison of human and animal mouth flora. *Journal of the Oklahoma State Medical Association* (1991), Vol 84, pp. 510-515.

the constant licking helps clear away dead tissue on a wound, which might help promote healing, but a dog's mouth is by no means "sterile" as some think. One study by Rayan and colleagues (1991) compared human and animal mouth flora; flora is the total amount of bacteria and other microorganisms in or on the body. Following their study, the authors concluded "Human oral flora contained the smallest number of bacteria followed by dog and cat oral flora, respectively." This seems logical, since most humans brush and floss their teeth once or twice a day, and, unlike humans, dogs will eat almost anything they find. However, many bacteria are species specific, so you're more likely to get sick if you kiss your son or daughter than if you kiss your puppy.

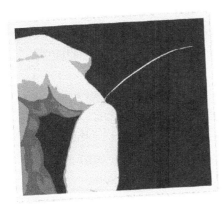

STRESS CAUSES HAIR TO TURN GRAY...

FALSE

HAVE YOU EVER heard someone say something like "you are going to give me gray hair" or "all this stress is going to turn me gray"? I actually remember saying this a few times in my life, for example when our children were progressing through the terrible twos. Well, there really is no scientific evidence that links stress and hair turning gray. Graying often starts in the mid thirties for Caucasians and the mid forties in people of color. However, graying can start as early as the mid to late teens or not start until a person's fifties or sixties. If you read much on this topic, you will likely come across the 50/50/50 principle. That is roughly fifty percent of people will have fifty percent of their hair turn gray by the time they are fifty years old. As I sit and write this chapter, I happen to be attending a meeting and am sitting directly behind a woman in her mid fifties. She has very long pretty hair, and I'd say that somewhere between fifty and sixty percent of her hair is gray.

Trueb, R. Aging of hair. *Journal of Cosmetic Dermatology* (2005), Vol 4, pp. 60-72.

I'm currently forty years old and started noticing the appearance of gray hairs five or six years ago, and it is progressing quickly! My father is in his mid seventies and has brilliantly white hair, so I anticipate that in the next five to ten years I will be completely gray. Some people work hard to cover up their gray hair with things like artificial coloring products whereas others just accept that graying is a normal part of the aging process. Some people even like to see their hair turn gray as they think it makes them look distinguished. What actually causes gray hair? Hair has the color it does due to a pigment called melanin. The cells that create melanin are called melanocytes. As we age, melanocytes die or produce less pigment, resulting in gray hair. An article (Trueb 2005) about aging hair also states that genetics play a role and autoimmune disorders can turn hair gray. Stress may be bad for your heart, but it won't turn your hair gray.

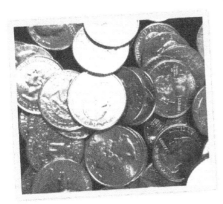

THE LONGER YOU SIT AT A SLOT MACHINE, THE GREATER YOUR ODDS ARE OF WINNING...

FALSE

IMAGINE THIS SCENARIO: you are in your favorite casino playing your favorite slot machine; you've been playing for about two and a half hours and just put your last quarter in hoping to hit it big. It didn't happen, and now you're out $125. You decide to head to the $19.95 all-you-can-eat buffet and drown your sorrows with BBQ ribs, fried chicken, and soft-serve ice cream. On your way to the buffet, you see the jackpot lights go off on the exact machine you just left. You think, if only I had stayed a couple of minutes longer, that jackpot would have been mine. The truth is that even if you would have stayed at the slot machine, you likely wouldn't have hit the jackpot. Today's slot machines use random number generators for the symbol combinations, so they are always changing; it is not possible to just "wait a machine out." If that were the case, you could just keep playing until you hit the jackpot. The truth is that the odds of hitting a jackpot on the third spin

Yucha, C., Bernhard, B., and Prato, C. Physiological effects of slot play in women. *Applied Psychophysiology and Biofeedback* (2007), Vol 32, pp. 141-147.

are the same as hitting a jackpot on the thirty thousandth spin. You also might think that if a machine hits a jackpot, it won't hit another one for some time. This is also not true. The odds are the same for hitting a jackpot on the very next spin. Many people find slot machines stimulating and fun to play. The authors of one study (Yucha 2007) reported that gambling increased physiological variables such as systolic and diastolic blood pressure, heart rate, respiratory rate, and skin temperature. It is understandable how people can get addicted to slots. However, if you're looking to actually win money at the casino, slots are not a very good bet. Your odds of winning at games like blackjack or craps are actually higher. Many slot machines are programmed to pay out roughly ninety-two percent, so for every dollar you put in, you win back on average ninety-two cents. Good deal for the casino; bad deal for you.

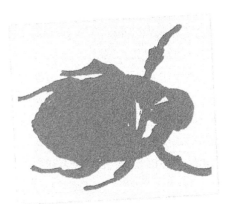

SOME RED FOOD COLORINGS ARE MADE FROM GROUND UP BUGS...

TRUE

THE NEXT TIME you pull out the red food coloring from your cupboard to make frosting for a cake, keep in mind that the food coloring may have been made from ground up bugs. The food colorings carmine and cochineal are in fact made from ground up insects—Dactylopius coccus bugs. These bugs live on opuntia cactus plants in South and Central America. When harvested and dried, roughly twenty percent of the volume of these insects is carminic acid; this is what is used to create food coloring. The bugs are harvested by scraping them off the cactus or collecting them in small baskets or nests attached to the cactus. It takes about seventy thousand bugs to make a pound of coloring! These particular food colorings are sometimes labeled as "natural coloring," "cochineal extract," "carmine," and "artificial coloring" on food labels. For obvious reasons, food manufacturing companies have made the decision to stay away from adding "crushed bugs" to their

Chung, K., Baker, J., Baldwin, J., and Chou, A. Identification of carmine allergens among three carmine allergy patients. *Allergy* (2001), Vol 56, pp. 73-77.

ingredients lists. These colorings were used by the Aztecs and other Indian populations in Mexico for a variety of reasons, such as coloring food and clothing. Today, cochineal extract and carmine can be found in products like yogurt, candy, fruit juices, and even cosmetics. These "natural" food colorings have increased in popularity over the past few years as some have suggested links between synthetic food dyes and cancer. The food colorings derived from bugs are generally considered to be safe; however, Chung, et al. (2001) report a number of cases of allergic reactions after individuals consumed carmine, and they reference other studies in their paper where carmine ingestion or exposure contributed to asthma, alveolitis, and food allergy. Understandably, certain cultures or groups of people are opposed to eating insects for religious or nutritional reasons, and then of course there is always the "eww" factor.

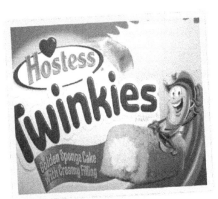

HOSTESS TWINKIES HAVE A SHELF LIFE OF JUST OVER TWO YEARS...

FALSE

AS I WAS preparing to write this chapter I realized it had been years since I'd enjoyed the sweet, spongy, cream filled delicacy that is the Twinkie. So I made my way to a store and soon realized I couldn't buy just one individual cake; I had to buy a box of ten. What I thought was going to cost me a quarter ended up costing me $3.39! Twinkies have been around since 1930 when a baker in Chicago wanted to better utilize shortcake pans and started experimenting with the cream-filled spongy cakes. Today there are about 500 million Twinkies made every year. The cakes were initially filled with a banana cream filling, but during WWII when bananas were hard to come by, the banana cream filling was replaced with a vanilla flavored filling. Many people think that Twinkies last a long time. I've heard people say they believe Twinkies have a shelf life of two, five, and even ten years. Some people even think that Twinkies never go bad because they are made from

Martins, R., Lopes, V., Vicente, A., and Teixeira, J. Computational shelf-life dating: Complex systems approaches to food quality and safety. *Food Bioprocessing Technology* (2008), Vol 1, pp. 207-222.

nothing but chemicals. Not true. The shelf life of Twinkies is about twenty-five days. The expiration date on my newly purchased Twinkies is March 1, and the day of purchase is February 16. In comparison, some MRE's (Meals Ready to Eat) can last up to ten years if stored at correct temperatures. Shelf life is defined as the time that a product is acceptable and meets the consumer's expectations regarding food quality (Martins 2008). Things that impact shelf life include temperature, water content, light exposure, and oxygen. There are a lot of chemicals in Twinkies (too many to list in this short chapter), but there is also flour, sugar, shortening, and eggs. If you indulge, do so in moderation as each cake contains 150 calories, 4.5 grams of fat, 27 grams of carbohydrates, and 220 mg of sodium.

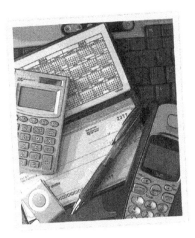

INDIVIDUALS WHO MULTITASK ARE MORE PRODUCTIVE...

FALSE

THERE HAS BEEN a fair amount of research performed on multitasking. However, before I reference a scientific study, I'd like to discuss an "informal experiment" I conducted with one of my best friends in a canoe on a sunny summer afternoon. My friend and I were fishing, and the fish were biting! My friend has the habit of using two or three rods at the same time, and this particular day he was using three. He held one in his hand, had one balanced in his lap, and had the other one propped up diagonally in the canoe. Not paying close attention to any of his rods, he missed many more fish than he caught. I'd estimate that I out-fished him five to one that afternoon. That was all the "evidence" I needed to confirm that it is better to focus on one task than to try and do multiple things at once. Our brains are wired in such a way that it is difficult for us to take in multiple streams of information at one time. Likewise, we are not wired to be able to perform more than

Ophir, E., Nass, C., and Wagner, A. Cognitive control in media multitaskers. *Psychological and Cognitive Sciences* (2009), Vol 106, pp. 15583-15587.

one task at a time very well. Try reading and saying the alphabet at the same time. Now you might think that, considering the lives many of us lead, multitasking seems to be a necessity. A vision of a mother paying the family bills, checking her son's homework, cooking dinner, answering e-mails, talking on the phone, all while listening to her iPod, comes to mind. The truth is that when we try to do two things at once, our productivity actually decreases. The authors of one study (Ophir, et al. 2009) which examined cognitive control in media multitaskers concluded, "This led to the surprising result that heavy media multitaskers performed worse on a test of task-switching ability." Not only can multitasking decrease productivity, but it can also be dangerous—think about the dangers of texting while driving!

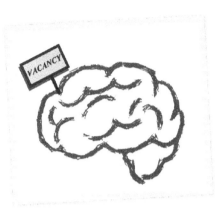

WE ONLY USE TEN PERCENT OF OUR BRAINS...

FALSE

IMAGINE IF YOU could take a supplement or complete a training program that would allow you to "unleash" the ninety percent of your brain that you currently don't use! The truth is that we really do use all of our brain. The ten percent myth has been circulating for many years. Lots of self-help gurus like us to think that we only use a small capacity of our brains because it enables them to sell a lot of products to us and make a lot of money. It is thought that famed psychologist William James may have inadvertently started this myth when he stated that humans only achieve a portion of their true potential. Somehow ten percent got attached to that statement, and it morphed into the myth that we only use ten percent of our brains. It is likely that the myth gained strength when it was mentioned in the preface of Dale Carnegie's book *How to Win Friends and Influence People*. For example, the authors of one study (Higbee 1998) performed on college students, a

Higbee, K. and Clay, S. College students' beliefs in the ten-percent myth. *The Journal of Psychology* (1998), Vol 132, pp. 469-476.

relatively well-educated population, reported that when participants were asked the question "About what percentage of their potential brain power do you think most people use?" over thirty-one percent of the students answered ten percent. Brain imaging scans have revealed that all parts of our brain are in fact active. We may use different portions of our brains for different functions, so different parts of our brains may be active at different times; however, there are no black holes or dead spaces in our brains. It is well documented in the medical literature that injury or damage to a small area of the brain can result in devastating neurological consequences. So rest assured that even on days when it doesn't seem like it, you are using all of your brain.

WOMEN TALK THREE TIMES AS MUCH AS MEN...

FALSE

IT IS A popular stereotype that women talk more than men. Many people think women talk a lot more, but very little conclusive research has been conducted on this topic. In 2006 Louann Brizendine published a book called *The Female Brain*. In it she wrote that women speak about twenty thousand words a day versus about seven thousand words a day for men. However, her claims were not supported by scientific studies. The only well-designed study I could find which examined the number of words spoken between men and women was conducted by Mehl and colleagues (2007) and published in the journal *Science*. The authors studied nearly four hundred college students over a seven year period. They used a device called an electronically activated recorder, EAR for short, to record words spoken throughout the day. The EAR device was set to record for thirty seconds every twelve and a half minutes that participants were awake (this averaged about seventeen

Mehl, M., Vazire, S., Ramirez-Esparaza, N., Slatcher, R., and Pennebaker, J. Are women really more talkative than men? *Science* (2007), Vol 317, p. 82.

hours a day). However, the device was set up in such a way so that the participants didn't know when the recording was taking place. When the study was completed, the authors learned that women spoke on average 16,215 words a day compared to 15,669 for men. So women did speak slightly more words per day but nowhere near thirteen thousand more. The fewest number of words spoken throughout the day was seven hundred, and the most was 47,000. The participant who spoke 47,000 words a day was a male! The authors did report that women talked more about other people and men talked more about concrete topics. If there is no scientific evidence that shows women speak more than men, how did this myth get so widespread? No one is really sure. One idea is that it originally came from marriage counselors, another from the notion that women often want to talk through their problems and men don't.

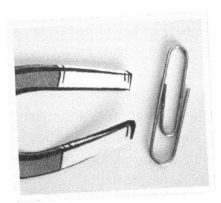

IT REALLY IS TRUE THAT OPPOSITES ATTRACT...

FALSE

WHEN MY WIFE and I met in college, I was immediately attracted to her beautiful smile and friendly personality. As we started to date, I realized that we were very different. She loved to read and could devour a book in a day or two; I usually read the minimum from my college textbooks to prepare for class and did no recreational reading. I was a bit of a sports fanatic; she likely couldn't have told you the difference between a touchdown and a home run. She enjoyed watching TV shows and movies with her friends, and I enjoyed ice fishing (we met in Minnesota) and walking through swamps pheasant and deer hunting. She was pretty laid back and didn't let things bother her too much; I had a mild case of obsessive compulsive disorder and a definite type A personality. I could fill this page with all the ways in which we were different from each other. Is that why we were initially attracted to each other—our differences? I'd like to think it was my rugged handsomeness,

Karney, B. and Bradbury, T. The longitudinal course of marriage quality and stability: A review of theory, method, and research. *Psychological Bulletin* (1995), Vol 118, pp. 3-34.

but that probably wasn't it. The topics of whether opposites attract and relational satisfaction have been well studied by researchers. Karney and Bradbury (1995) published a review article in which they examined many studies on marriage. In the article the authors state that greater attitude and personality homogamy (similarity) between spouses predicts greater marital stability and satisfaction. Studies have also shown that even in the early stages of meeting and dating someone, we tend to be more attracted to people similar to us (think of the saying 'birds of a feather flock together'). The same holds true for our friendships; we like to be around people who like the same things we do. No one is really sure where this myth came from, but we often hear of the good girl falling for the bad boy, and we frequently see this scenario (opposites attracting) in movie plots.

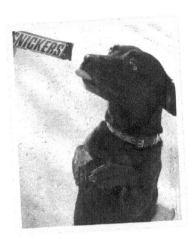

CHOCOLATE IS VERY HARMFUL TO DOGS AND CAN EVEN KILL THEM...

TRUE

YEARS AGO MY wife and I took a leisurely stroll with our beloved dog, Cody. The walk was uneventful until Cody came to a dead stop that nearly pulled my arm out of its socket. Since he wasn't doing his doggy duty, I closely inspected my pet to learn the reason for his odd behavior. I discovered that he had found a perfectly intact chocolate bon bon on the ground, and was holding it gently in his mouth, head down, indicating that he knew full well that it was forbidden. To make a long story short, my wife was panicked, certain that Cody would die on the spot, and Cody was just as desperate to keep his prize. Amazingly, the dog actually forfeited the chocolate after much coaxing and lived to see another day. While one bon bon likely wouldn't have killed Cody, it is true that chocolate is harmful to dogs and can result in serious health problems or possibly even death. The authors of a short article which appeared in the *British Medical Journal* (2005) wrote, "The potential hazards

Finlay, F. and Guiton, S. Chocolate poisoning. *British Medical Journal* (2005), Vol 331, p. 633.

to humans of eating too much chocolate are well known (obesity and dental caries to name but two), but you may be unaware that chocolate is potentially lethal to dogs." There is a chemical in chocolate called theobromine, and this is what is so harmful to dogs. Different types of chocolates contain different amounts of theobromine, however. White chocolate contains very little theobromine and is usually not considered to be harmful to canines. Milk chocolate contains sixty milligrams per ounce, semisweet chocolate 160 milligrams per ounce, and bakers chocolate about 450 milligrams per ounce. Consuming theobromine will likely stimulate a dog's central nervous system and heart as well as increase its blood pressure. Additional negative effects could include vomiting, diarrhea, muscle spasms, excessive panting, and increased urination. If you have a dog that consumes chocolate, the best thing to do is to call your veterinarian immediately.

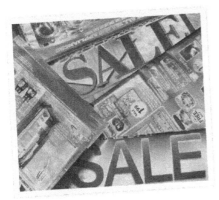

THE BIGGEST SHOPPING DAY OF THE YEAR IS THE DAY AFTER THANKSGIVING...

FALSE

THE FRIDAY FOLLOWING Thanksgiving is known as Black Friday. Many consider this day to be the "official" beginning of the holiday shopping season. It is common for stores to run huge promotions on Black Friday, sometimes slashing prices on large ticket items to get shoppers into stores. I'm someone who loves to read the paper and have a few too many cups of coffee in the morning. I'm always amazed by the size and weight of the paper the morning after Thanksgiving, due to the flyers and advertisements alerting potential shoppers of the deals that await them. It is also common to see news stories focusing on the hoards of shoppers often lined up in front of stores at 4:00 or 5:00 a.m. waiting for the doors to open so that they can get their deals. Regretfully, we also hear about fights, injuries and, less commonly, even deaths associated with Black Friday. In 2008 an employee at a Wal-Mart was trampled to death as shoppers broke through the

http://www.snopes.com/holidays/thanksgiving/shopping.asp. Website accessed April 23, 2010.

store's doors before the scheduled opening time. With all the attention given to Black Friday, it is easy to see why people might think it is the biggest shopping day of the year. Snopes. com, an urban legend reference page which is widely known for debunking myths and misconceptions, reports that Black Friday may be the day the greatest number of shoppers are visiting retail stores and shopping malls, but it is not the biggest shopping day in regard to dollars spent. Traditionally, the day shoppers spend the most money is the Saturday before Christmas. I have to confess, that is the day I usually do ALL of my Christmas shopping, alongside many other people! So why the term Black Friday? Supposedly the term started to be used in Philadelphia in the 1960's to describe the increased number of people and cars on the streets following Thanksgiving Day. However, it is also often reported in the media that the term refers to the day that stores start to turn a profit (get into the black) in regard to their sales.

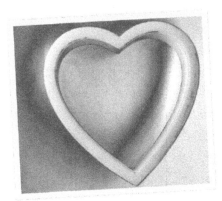

MORE CANDY IS SOLD FOR VALENTINE'S DAY THAN ANY OTHER HOLIDAY...

FALSE

VALENTINE'S DAY, ANOTHER opportunity for me to forget a "special" occasion for my wife and be riddled with guilt. As if remembering to buy gifts on Christmas, birthdays, Easter, anniversaries, ground hog's day, mother's day, and of course helping my kids pull off an April Fools prank isn't enough! Valentine's Day, celebrated on February 14th, was established in AD 500 and has traditionally been a day for lovers to display affection for each other by offering gifts of cards, candy, and flowers. It is thought that the designation "Valentine's Day" came from a Christian martyr or martyrs named Valentine. According to the website of the National Confectioners Association (NCA), one of those men, a priest named Valentine, was beheaded by order of the Roman emperor Claudius II on February 14th 270 AD because he was performing marriage ceremonies, something the emperor had outlawed. The website also says that more than

Echeandia, J. Candy review: Holiday candy sales insights courtesy of Hershey Company; Seasonal candy sales for 2007 grew at Valentine and Easter in spite of short selling seasons. *Confectioner* (May 2007).

36 million boxes of heart shaped candy are sold for Valentine's Day. Another tradition related to Valentine's Day, in no way connected to lovers, is for children to exchange valentines at school. Our three children usually come home with dozens of valentines, and most of them have heart shaped candy, a sucker, or some form of cavity-causing delicacy attached to them. It's really no surprise, then, that so many people think more candy is sold for Valentine's Day than any other holiday. The truth is, however, that Valentine's Day ranks fourth on the list of holidays for candy purchases. According to sales figures for 2007 compiled by the National Confectioners Association based upon data from Information Resources, Inc., and cited in an article published in *Confectioner* (2007), the top four selling holidays for candy were Valentine's Day (1 billion), Christmas (1.4 billion), Easter (1.9 billion) and Halloween (2.1 billion). Trick or treat!

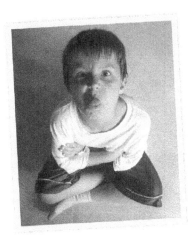

"ONLY" CHILDREN ARE MORE SELFISH, BOSSY, AND SPOILED...

FALSE

MYTH 87

IT IS A common misconception that only children (sometimes referred to as "onlies") are spoiled, selfish, and rotten little brats. To most people it makes perfect sense, and it may even be somewhat logical. When parents have only one child, that child gets all the attention, all the toys, all the affection, and all the coolest birthday presents; they don't even have any competition selecting which cartoons they are going to watch on Saturday morning. How could they not be self-centered? There has been tremendous growth in the number of single child family units in the past five to ten years. There has also been a fair amount of research looking into whether only children are indeed spoiled and selfish compared to other children with siblings. It appears that they are not. Mancillas (2006) published a very good review article on the topic in the *Journal of Counseling and Development* stating, "There is clearly a need to correct the negative bias and stereotypes

Mancillas, A. Challenging the stereotypes about only children: A review of the literature and implications for practice. *Journal of Counseling and Development* (2006), Vol 84, pp. 268-275.

181

about only children, not only to benefit children and families but to ensure that mental health professionals, researchers, educators, and policy makers articulate an accurate understanding of only children and their families..." Many children are spoiled and bossy at various times in their lives. I'm a father of three children, and I have to say that it has been my experience that children (at least mine—and all my friends' children) at some point think everything should revolve around them. This commonly happens in a child's early years, but I've also heard that this can be the case during the teenage years as well, as shocking as that may sound. Everything I've ever read and been taught suggests that how a child acts and behaves is much more a result of parenting style than number of siblings or birth order.

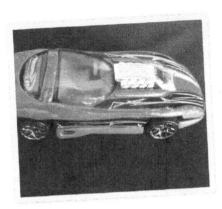

PEOPLE WHO DRIVE RED CARS GET PULLED OVER MORE OFTEN...

FALSE

EVERY TIME MY wife and I contemplate buying a different vehicle, we spend a lot of time walking around car dealerships and examining our many options. The first thing I usually notice when looking for a new car is the price tag. My reaction is often one of sheer horror—followed by disbelief—and this question: can that really be the correct price for this vehicle? Shortly after the sticker shock wears off, I take a good look at the color and ask myself: is this a color I can tolerate for the next five or even ten years? Inevitably, we come to a shiny red car and I have to sit in it, just for fun. I've always believed the old saying that red cars get pulled over more often for speeding. Just sitting idly in the showroom, they look fast. It turns out that there has not been a lot of research examining whether the color of vehicles impacts the frequency at which the drivers of those vehicles get stopped and/or ticketed. However, the little research that is available suggests that this

Newman, M. and Willis, F. Bright cars and speeding tickets. *Journal of Applied Social Psychology* (1993), Vol 23, pp. 79-83.

is just an old wives' tale or urban legend. Newman and Willis (1993) conducted the only published study I could find looking at car color and the chance of getting a speeding ticket. These authors monitored speeding tickets over a twenty-two month period and compared the frequency of tickets by car color to the frequency of cars on the road with those colors. They found that red cars get ticketed about the same amount as gray and brown cars. About ninety-five percent of the tickets in this study were the result of using radar, and many times when radar is used the speed is already obtained before an officer notices the color of the car. Some think that red cars give the appearance of going faster; there really is no good scientific evidence for this either. So go ahead and buy the bright shiny red car without fear of being pulled over and ticketed more often.

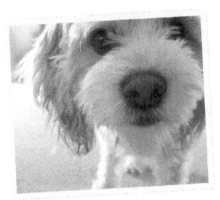

CERTAIN DOGS CAN SMELL CANCER...

TRUE

MANY PEOPLE AFFECTIONATELY refer to dogs as man's best friend. I've grown up with dogs and have always had dogs in my life, so I would wholeheartedly agree with that statement. Dogs provide us with companionship, help seeing-impaired individuals safely navigate streets and sidewalks, and help farmers and ranchers herd sheep and cattle; dogs are also used to locate missing persons and detect things like drugs and bombs (a dog's sense of smell is estimated to be 10,000 to 100,000 times more sensitive than a human's). Recently, I had a chance to spend some time with a gentleman (Mike) from England at an outdoor archery range. Mike happened to have epilepsy and always traveled with his dog. I learned that day that Mike's dog could warn Mike before he was going to have a seizure. Usually the warning (barking) came two to five hours before a seizure occurred, and Mike said his dog was right one hundred percent of the time. I was truly amazed!

McCulloch, M., Jezierski, T., Broffman, M., Hubbard, A., Turner, K., and Janecki, T. Diagnostic accuracy of canine scent detection in early- and late-stage lung and breast cancers. *Integrative Cancer Therapies* (2006), Vol 5, pp. 30-39.

It now appears that dogs may also start being used to help detect cancer. A study by McCulloch and colleagues (2006) published in the journal *Integrative Cancer Therapies* examined whether dogs could be trained to detect cancer simply by sniffing someone's breath. Due to increased oxidative stress, cancer cells emit slightly different waste products than normal cells. The results of the study suggest that dogs can be trained to smell cancer with high degrees of sensitivity and specificity. The authors concluded that "training was efficient and cancer identification was accurate; in a matter of weeks, ordinary household dogs with only basic behavioral 'puppy training' were trained to accurately distinguish breath samples of lung and breast cancer patients from those of controls." The dogs used for the study were Portuguese water dogs and Labrador retrievers, but the ability to be trained to detect cancer is probably not breed specific.

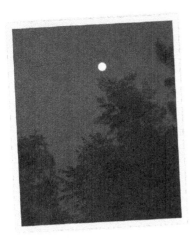

THERE IS A LINK BETWEEN THE FULL MOON AND BAD BEHAVIOR IN HUMANS...

FALSE

MYTH 90

IF I WERE to base my response to this myth on what occurs in television shows and movies, the answer would be a resounding "yes!" TV shows and movies frequently have werewolves, zombies, and many other undesirables coming out during a full moon to engage in their sinister activities. These media outlets also exaggerate the amount of crime and abnormal human behavior that occurs during a full moon. This idea that the moon triggers a wide variety of deviant behavior in humans has been with us for many years. Consider that lunacy, which means insanity, is derived from the Latin word "luna" for moon. The full moon is frequently associated with or blamed for things like murder and other crimes, alcoholism, epilepsy, arson, natural disasters, suicide, and mental illness. It is also common for people to think that the moon influences things like the weather, fertility, and birthrates. We frequently read about police officers, paramedics, nurses, and

Rotton, J. and Kelly, I. Much ado about the full moon: A meta-analysis of lunar-lunacy research. *Psychological Bulletin* (1985), Vol 97, pp. 286-306.

physicians believing that crime rates increase and emergency room visits skyrocket during periods of a full moon. However, this belief is not supported by scientific studies. A few of the many studies that have been conducted on this topic have shown a relationship or association between the full moon and bad behavior, but the overwhelming evidence suggests there is no correlation between the two. Rotton and Kelly (1985) reviewed thirty-seven studies on this topic in an article published in the journal *Psychological Bulletin* and stated, "Although this meta-analysis uncovered a few statistically significant relations between phases of the moon and behavior, it cannot be concluded that people behave any more (or less) strangely during one phase of the moon than another." Again, most of the studies conducted and published do not support the idea that the full moon influences human behavior in any way whatsoever.

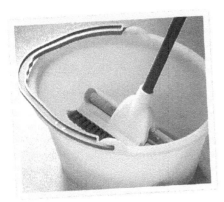

HAVING A HUSBAND CREATES SEVEN EXTRA HOURS OF HOUSEWORK A WEEK FOR WOMEN...

TRUE

IT'S TRUE! HAVING a husband does create an extra seven hours of housework each week for women. I have to admit I'm feeling a tinge of guilt as I sit and write these words. I've been scolded so many times for walking through the house with my shoes on that I'm surprised I still have shoes. I'll also admit to having done the dishes a few times without using soap and throwing light and dark colored clothes together in the same load of laundry with the hope that everything would not turn pink. Now, my wife cringes if I even get near the sink or the washing machine. I still get to take out the trash, pick up after the dog, and do most of the weeding in the garden, however. A research study directed by economist Frank Stafford at the University of Michigan Institute for Social Research revealed that women sweep, dust, mop, clean, and pick up an average of seven hours more each week because of their husbands. On the other hand, having a wife saves husbands roughly an hour

Public release date 4-4-2008 http://www.eurekalert.org/pub_releases/2008-04/uom-ehm040408.php.

of housework a week. It's interesting how much research has been done on who does the household chores. It really isn't as simple as it was sixty or seventy years ago when more women stayed home and the expectation was that they would take care of much of the housework. Today, with many more dual income families, couples have to work together and decide who is going to do the laundry, cleaning, cooking, and tidying up. The study directed by Stafford revealed some interesting trends. Overall, women spend less time doing housework today (seventeen hours a week) compared to 1976 (twenty-six hours a week) whereas men do more than double the housework today (thirteen hours a week) compared to 1976 (six hours a week). The study also revealed that younger single women (in their twenties and thirties) did the least amount of housework a week, about twelve hours, and married women with more than three children did the most, about twenty-eight hours a week.

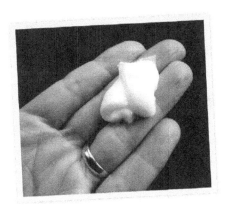

COCOA BUTTER ELIMINATES STRETCH MARKS...

FALSE

STRETCH MARKS (THE medical name is striae gravidarum) are those linear scar-looking lines that appear on the skin. They commonly appear on the stomach and breasts but can also appear on the legs and buttocks. They are frequently a dark purple in color and are a source of embarrassment for many. Stretch marks sometimes appear following pregnancy, after large gains in muscle mass in weight lifters and body builders, or other significant weight gains in a relatively short time period. I experienced stretch marks my freshman year in college when I gained fifty pounds after just nine months (unlimited meal plan in the cafeteria). My wife also developed stretch marks following the birth of our first child. Interestingly, both of us were informed by healthcare providers that using cocoa butter would help eliminate stretch marks and would help prevent more stretch marks from occurring in the future.

Osman, H., Usta, I., Rubeiz, N., Abu-Rustum, R., Charara, I., and Nassar, A. Cocoa butter lotion for prevention of striae gravidarum: A double blind, randomized and placebo-controlled trial. *International Journal of Obstetrics and Gynaecology* (2008), Vol 115, pp. 1138-1142.

We both tried cocoa butter but didn't notice any change in the appearance of the marks. After performing a quick internet search I came across many sites that promote the use of cocoa butter for stretch marks, but the claims of what cocoa butter could do were never backed up by scientific evidence. I was able to find one study (Osman, et al. 2008) where researchers randomly assigned pregnant women to a group that received lotion containing cocoa butter and another group of pregnant women to a group that received a placebo lotion that did not contain cocoa butter. The women entered the study during the first trimester of pregnancy and were instructed to apply the lotion until delivery. Following the study there was no difference in the development of stretch marks in the women who used cocoa butter lotion and those who didn't. The authors concluded that their findings did not support the use of cocoa butter lotion to prevent stretch marks.

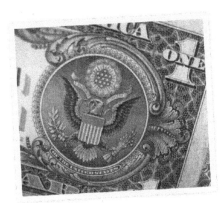

YOU SPEND LESS MONEY WHEN YOU USE CASH VS. CREDIT CARDS...

TRUE

ACCORDING TO THE website Creditcards.com, the average credit card debt in households that use credit cards is over $15,000, and there are over 500 million credit cards in circulation in the U.S. I knew that credit card debt was a problem for many people, but I didn't realize just how big the problem was. If you own and use credit cards, you in all honesty can probably answer the question of whether you spend more money when using credit cards vs. using cash. My wife and I stopped using credit cards years ago. We never had a problem with carrying credit card debt, but we noticed that we spent roughly twenty to twenty-five percent more money when we made purchases with our credit cards vs. using cash. There have been a few research studies conducted on this topic, and most show that you indeed spend more money when you use credit cards, roughly eight to eighteen percent more. One early study was conducted by Elizabeth Hirschman

Hirschman, E. Differences in consumer purchase behavior by credit card payment system. *Journal of Consumer Research* (1979), Vol 6, pp. 58-66.

(1979) and published in the *Journal of Consumer Research*. Dr. Hirschman hypothesized that consumers who only had bank- or store-issued cards would make larger total dollar purchases than those not possessing a card and that the average transaction with a card would be higher than transactions made with cash. The results of the study supported her hypotheses and showed that consumers did indeed spend more money and also made more purchases when using cards. One reason we might spend more money using credit cards is that it is much easier to make spontaneous purchases. Many years ago when my wife and I still had our credit cards, we were walking through a sporting goods store and happened past the firearms area. I'm still not sure how it happened, but in a matter of twenty minutes we purchased two firearms with the total bill being over a thousand dollars. We likely would not have made that purchase if we hadn't had our credit cards in our wallets.

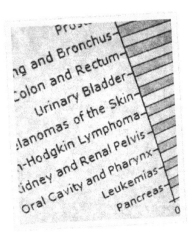

CANCER RATES HAVE INCREASED DRAMATICALLY OVER THE PAST TEN YEARS...

FALSE

MYTH 94

CANCER IS A disease whereby cells divide and grow abnormally, often spreading throughout the body and invading other organs and tissues. According to the National Cancer Institute (NCI), there are over one hundred different types of cancers with the main categories being 1) carcinoma, 2) sarcoma, 3) leukemia, 4) lymphoma and myeloma, and 5) central nervous system cancers. Most people know someone who has battled or is currently battling cancer. It is not surprising that most people mistakenly believe that cancer rates are on the rise, but just the opposite is true. The National Cancer Institute's *Cancer Trends Progress Report* for 2009/2010 reveals that death rates for lung, breast, prostate, and colorectal cancers, the four cancers that occur the most frequently, are on the decline. In fact, death rates for all cancers combined continue to go down. The report indicates that the number of people getting cancer has continued to go down

National Cancer Institute, U.S. National Institutes of Health. *Cancer Trends Progress Report–2009/2010* Update. http://progressreport.cancer.gov/. Accessed July 21, 2010.

since about 2000. Historically speaking, the incidence of cancer increased from the mid 1970's to about 1990, then leveled off for the next ten years or so, and has been on the decline since. It is important to note that rates for some cancers are on the rise. Those would include esophagus, pancreas, liver, bile duct, testis, kidney, leukemia, thyroid, melanoma of the skin, and childhood cancer. Cancer is the second leading cause of death in the United States; heart disease is the first. The Centers for Disease Control and Prevention reported that in 2007, 616,067 people died of heart disease and 562,875 people died of cancer. The NCI report also stated that blacks had the highest rate of new cancers, followed by whites, with lower rates for Hispanics and Asians. If you want to try and reduce your risk of getting cancer, avoid smoking, eat a healthy balanced diet, engage in regular physical activity, and maintain a normal weight.

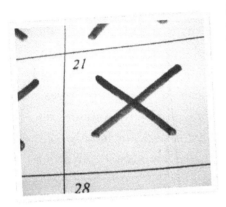

IT TAKES 21 DAYS TO DEVELOP OR BREAK A HABIT...

MYTH 95

FALSE

MOST OF US have habits we would like to change or can think of things we should be doing more consistently to improve our lives. Some of us would like to quit smoking, maybe become more active, eat more fruits and vegetables, floss our teeth on a regular basis, or even turn the television off and challenge our children to a game of chess. It's a common belief that if you can change a behavior for twenty-one days, it will likely stick. Just for fun, as I often do, I searched the internet to see what was out there on this topic. I came across this from someone who really believes it takes twenty-one days to develop a habit: "In order to ensure behavior change, experts agree that it takes a minimum of twenty-one days to change a behavior." The "to ensure" and "experts agree" portions of this statement were very interesting. I immediately thought of my father, who quit smoking cold turkey after thirty years of smoking one to two packs of cigarettes a day. He changed his

Webb, T., Sheeran, P., and Luszczynska, A. Planning to break unwanted habits: Habit strength moderates implementation intention effects on behavior change. *British Journal of Social Psychology* (2009), Vol 48, pp. 507-523.

behavior in a day and has never smoked since; that was about thirty years ago. I also think of many friends and acquaintances who were able to stop smoking, drinking, or gambling for more than twenty-one days only to fall back into their old addictive behaviors, sometimes even after months or years had gone by. Most of us know individuals who start an exercise program and do it religiously for weeks or months, only to eventually fall back into their sedentary lifestyle. An article by Webb and colleagues (2009) on breaking unwanted habits explored some strategies for changing unwanted behaviors; it also mentions factors that might make breaking those habits more difficult. I could find no reference, however, to the idea of its taking twenty-one days to either develop or break a habit in this article or any of the other scientific articles I reviewed.

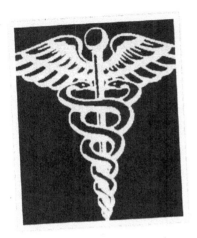

MEDICAL ERRORS IN HOSPITALS KILL MORE PEOPLE PER YEAR THAN CAR ACCIDENTS...

TRUE

I GENERALLY DON'T take an alarmist approach to the topics I cover and write about, and I have to admit that I've not thought much about complications and deaths caused by the errors of physicians, nurses, and other health care professionals. However, since the Institute of Medicine (IOM) released a report in 1999 entitled *To Err Is Human: Building A Safer Health System*, it seems that more people are taking a closer look at this topic. The IOM report stated that at least 44,000 people, and perhaps as many as 98,000 people, die in hospitals each year as a result of medical errors that could have been prevented. In contrast, National Highway Traffic Safety Administration statistics show that in 2008, 34,017 people died in motor vehicle accidents. The IOM report defined medical errors as the failure of a planned action to be completed as intended or the use of a wrong plan to achieve an aim, and claimed that these errors cost the country

Kohn, L., Corrigan, J., and Donaldson, M., eds. *To Err Is Human: Building a Safer Health System.* Washington, DC: National Academy Press, 1999.

seventeen to twenty-nine billion dollars annually. It's hard to imagine that in a country as advanced as the United States so many deaths are attributed to medical errors in hospitals. When most people think about the health care system in the U.S., they generally think that it is one of the best systems in the world. However, organizations that rank health care systems from various countries don't show that to be the case. For example, the World Health Organization has ranked the U.S.'s health care system thirty-seventh out of 191 countries. Medical errors can be attributed to sloppy handwriting, lack of communication among healthcare providers, inappropriately prescribed dosages of medication, and many other scenarios. To help reduce the chance of a medial error occurring to you, make sure that you communicate well with your physician, get all your health related-questions answered, and get a second opinion if you are not feeling comfortable with the advice you are being given.

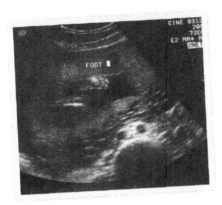

THE TIMING OF CONCEPTION OFTEN DETERMINES THE GENDER OF YOUR BABY...

MYTH 97

FALSE

I THINK IT'S interesting that some couples try so hard to influence the potential gender of their children. There are supposedly lots of things that can impact whether conception results in a boy or a girl being born. The Chinese have a gender selection chart, or calendar, which suggests that conception occurring on certain days of the year will result in either male or female babies being born. Other possibilities include selecting certain positions during intercourse, eating certain types of foods, and even sleeping in certain positions. Medical personnel agree that the gender of a child is determined when a single sperm cell fertilizes an egg. The egg always carries an X chromosome while a single sperm can carry either an X (girl) or Y (boy) chromosome. So if a sperm cell that fertilizes an egg is carrying an X chromosome, a girl will be the conceived whereas a boy will be conceived if the sperm cell that fertilizes an egg is carrying the Y chromosome. Studies

Wilcox, A., Weinberg, C., and Baird, D. Timing of sexual intercourse in relation to ovulation: Effects on the probability of conception, survival of the pregnancy, and sex of the baby. *New England Journal of Medicine* (1995), Vol 333, pp. 1517-1521.

have shown that sperm with a Y chromosome (boys) are faster swimmers, but are not as strong and don't live as long as sperm with an X chromosome. If you consider that conception usually occurs close to ovulation (most estimate a two to ten day range), it would stand to reason that timing could be a factor. For example, if intercourse occurs further away from ovulation, the sperm with the girl chromosome would likely have the advantage, due to a longer lifespan. However, this is not supported in the medical literature. The authors of one study published in the *New England Journal of Medicine* (1995) examined this topic and reported, "However, we found no association between the sex of the baby and timing of intercourse in relation to ovulation. We conclude that the deliberate timing of intercourse around the day of ovulation has no practical value in sex selection."

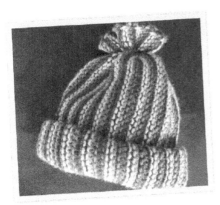

YOU LOSE MORE HEAT THROUGH YOUR HEAD THAN ANY OTHER PART OF YOUR BODY...

FALSE

I REGULARLY HEAR people talk about how we should keep our heads covered when we are in the cold because we lose lots of heat through our heads. I've heard numbers like fifty or even as much as seventy-five percent of the heat we lose is lost through our heads. The head makes up roughly eight to ten percent of the total surface area of the body, and heat loss through the head usually accounts for roughly eight or nine percent of the total amount of heat we lose. An interesting trend of late is men with any sign of hair loss or balding completely shaving their heads. When you see a shaved, completely bald and rounded shiny head, I can see how you might think that this would be an easy way for heat to leave the body. However, when we are in cold environments we will lose heat from any exposed areas of our bodies; the heat loss is about the same whether it comes from the head, arms, torso, or legs. It is true that the head and scalp have a very healthy blood

Pretorius, T., Bristow, G., Steinman, A., and Giesbrecht, G. Thermal effects of whole head submersion in cold water on nonshivering humans. *Journal of Applied Physiology* (2006), Vol 101, pp. 669-675.

supply; you've probably realized that if you've ever had a laceration or cut on your head or face—lots of blood! This might be one of the reasons that people think we proportionally lose more heat from our heads. Other reasons might include some early flawed military studies and statements about excessive heat loss through our heads in an army survival manual. One way researchers study this is to immerse participants' heads in cold water and monitor body temperature. In a study by Bristow and colleagues (2006) published in the *Journal of Applied Physiology*, the authors state, "In conclusion, whole head submersion in seventeen degree water did not contribute relatively more than the rest of the body to total surface heat loss." Ultimately, it's not a bad idea to keep your head covered when you are out in the cold because it might help keep your ears from getting frostbitten, but remember that you don't lose more heat through your head compared to other parts of your body.

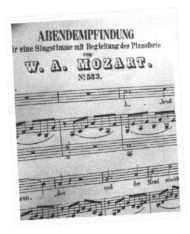

HAVING BABIES LISTEN TO MOZART WILL MAKE THEM SMARTER...

FALSE

MYTH 99

BEING PARENTS OF three children, I can tell you that my wife and I have had many of the same concerns and worries that millions of parents have had regarding their children's intelligence and academic abilities. Why isn't my child talking yet? When will she start reading? How are my child's writing and math skills compared to their playmates? Should we send our child to an expensive private pre-school program? Is there anything else we can do to help "speed things up" academically for our children and give them that competitive edge as they take that monumental and daunting leap into kindergarten? I also remember considering playing classical music to our children when they were young because we had heard that it improves intelligence, something referred to as the Mozart effect. We didn't opt for the expensive pre-schools and we didn't make our kids listen to Mozart, and academically speaking they are doing just fine. The hype surrounding

Pietschnig, J., Voracek, M., and Formann, A. Mozart effect – Shmozart effect: A meta-analysis. *Intelligence* (2010), Vol 38, pp. 314-323.

the Mozart effect, which now has a whole industry surrounding it with dozens of products and tens of millions of dollars in sales, started after a study on college students done in the early 1990's showed that they performed better on a spatial reasoning task, a test where they had to fold and cut paper, after they listened to Mozart for ten minutes. Interestingly, this initial study did not include children or tests of intelligence. Many studies have since disproved the Mozart effect. Pietschnig and colleagues (2010) published a meta-analysis of dozens of studies that have been done to date and concluded that "in summary, this study shows that there is little support for a Mozart effect considering the cumulative empirical evidence." In other words, exposing your children to Mozart or other classical music when they are in the womb, two months old, or two years old, will likely not increase their intelligence.

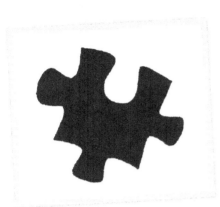

THERE HAS BEEN A TREMENDOUS INCREASE IN AUTISM RATES RECENTLY...

FALSE

THINKING BACK TO my childhood, I can't remember ever hearing the word autism or having a friend who was autistic. Today, however, most of us, even our children, know someone who has been diagnosed with autism. Gernsbacher and colleagues (2005) in an article published in the journal *Current Directions in Psychological Science* state that autism was first described as a standalone disorder in the 1940's, but it wasn't until 1980 that criteria for autism was included in the American Psychiatric Associations' Diagnostic and Statistical Manual of Mental Disorders. The CDC describes autism spectrum disorders (ASD's) as a group of disorders that can result in social, communication, and behavioral challenges. The "spectrum" in ASD's indicates that the impact the disorder can have on an individual could be minor, or it could be very severe. The prevalence of autism appeared to dramatically increase in the early to mid 1990's; however, it wasn't

Gernsbacher, M., Dawson, M., and Goldsmith, H. Three reasons not to believe in an autism epidemic. *Current Directions in Psychological Science* (2005), Vol 14, pp. 55-58.

clear if the increase was due to actual new cases of autism or increases in diagnosis and reporting. Some believe that Thimerosal, a mercury-containing compound in vaccines, is responsible for the increase in autism rates. However, there appears to be a lack of scientific evidence to connect the two. Additionally, in the article referenced above, Gernsbacher and colleagues discuss a variety of reasons they believe there has not been an epidemic of autism recently. The authors state that "no sound scientific evidence indicates that the increasing number of diagnosed cases of autism arise from anything other than purposely broadened diagnostic criteria, coupled with deliberately greater public awareness, and intentionally improved case finding." So it appears that there truly has not been a dramatic increase in autism rates recently, simply changes in diagnostic criteria and public awareness.

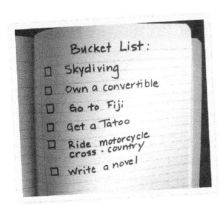

Bucket List:

☐ Skydiving
☐ Own a convertible
☐ Go to Fiji
☐ Get a Tatoo
☐ Ride motorcycle cross-country
☐ Write a novel

MOST PEOPLE EXPERIENCE A MID-LIFE CRISIS...

FALSE

WE OFTEN HEAR stories of individuals in their 40's or 50's who go through drastic life changes. Sometimes it's a decision to get divorced, change jobs, move across the country, or maybe buy a sports car or even better a Harley Davidson. Often the explanation or blame for these behaviors falls to the individual having a mid-life crisis. Supposedly, many things can lead to someone's having a mid-life crisis; some of the possibilities include unhappiness with a spouse, a lack of meaning or direction in one's life, a feeling of unfulfilled goals or dreams, menopause, or simply a desire for fun, excitement, and adventure. I think it's safe to say that many of the things that supposedly lead to a mid-life crisis regularly occur to people when they are in their 20's or 30's and even their 60's or 70's. I was unable to uncover any research that specifically described when a mid-life crisis usually started, how long it usually lasts, or the best way to get out of one should

Charles, S., Reynolds, C., and Gatz, M. Age-related differences and change in positive and negative affect over 23 years. *Journal of Personality and Social Psychology* (2001), Vol 80, pp. 136-151.

it occur. A study published in the *Journal of Personality and Social Psychology* by Reynolds, et al. (2001) suggests that as we get older positive affect, things like joy and excitement, remain fairly stable whereas negative affect, things like anger, disgust, anguish, and shame, actually decreases. The authors also discuss how additional research findings don't support the idea that middle age is a time when many people go into crisis mode. They cite some studies showing that differences in life satisfaction change little across the lifespan and also discuss how some research actually supports the idea of greater well-being in older adults. While some people may go through hard times during the mid-life years, this is often the time when people are getting promoted, earning a decent salary, happily raising children, and generally feeling pretty good about themselves.

ABOUT THE AUTHOR

BRIAN UDERMANN is a Full Professor in the Department of Exercise and Sport Science and also serves as the Director of Online Education at the University of Wisconsin-La Crosse. He earned his Bachelor's degree in Sports Medicine from St. Cloud State University, and earned both his Masters (Health and Physical Education) and Doctoral (Science Education/ Exercise Physiology) degrees from Syracuse University. Research interests include health and wellness, myths and misconceptions, teaching effectiveness, online education, low back pain, and the effect of spirituality on health and healing. His research has been presented at national and international conferences which include The Hawaiian International Conference on Education, The National Athletic Trainers' Association's Educators' Conference, The International Society for the Study of the Lumbar Spine, and The American College of Sports Medicine. Brian has over forty national and international presentations, has published five book chapters and roughly fifty peer reviewed manuscripts in scholarly journals. His research appears in such journals as *The Athletic Training Education Journal*, T*he Journal of Online Learning* and Teaching, *The Journal of Sports Sciences and Medicine, The Journal of Athletic Training, Archives of Physical Medicine and Rehabilitation, The Journal of Back and Musculoskeletal Rehabilitation, The Journal of Strength and Conditioning Research, The Clinical Journal of Sports Medicine, Research Quarterly for Exercise and Sport, The Physician and Sports Medicine,* and the *Spine Journal.* Brian frequently speaks on the topic of myths and misconceptions; please contact him if you are interested in scheduling a presentation.

I TRULY ENJOY writing about myths and want to continue to do so. If you can think of a myth that you would like to have seen included in this book, please contact me and let me know what it is. I'm a strong advocate of getting feedback on the work I do and continually work to make improvements. If there were things you enjoyed about this book, I would very much like to know about them; conversely, if there are things you didn't enjoy about this book or if you can think of things I could do to improve future books, I would appreciate knowing what those are as well. I will try hard to respond to each communication I receive. Also, please feel free to visit my website at www.isynergikeynotes.com, which contains an area called "Myth of the Week." If you would like to be contacted each week when a new myth is added, simply send me your name and e-mail address so that I can add you to the list.

Thank you!

BRIAN UDERMANN
e-mail: brian@isynergikeynotes.com
Phone: 608.386.0108

INDEX